STUDIES IN IMPERIALISM

General editor: Andrew S. Thompson
Founding editor: John M. MacKenzie

When the 'Studies in Imperialism' series was founded by Professor John M. MacKenzie more than thirty years ago, emphasis was laid upon the conviction that 'imperialism as a cultural phenomenon had as significant an effect on the dominant as on the subordinate societies'. With well over a hundred titles now published, this remains the prime concern of the series. Cross-disciplinary work has indeed appeared covering the full spectrum of cultural phenomena, as well as examining aspects of gender and sex, frontiers and law, science and the environment, language and literature, migration and patriotic societies, and much else. Moreover, the series has always wished to present comparative work on European and American imperialism, and particularly welcomes the submission of books in these areas. The fascination with imperialism, in all its aspects, shows no sign of abating, and this series will continue to lead the way in encouraging the widest possible range of studies in the field. 'Studies in Imperialism' is fully organic in its development, always seeking to be at the cutting edge, responding to the latest interests of scholars and the needs of this ever-expanding area of scholarship.

Venomous encounters

MANCHESTER
1824

Manchester University Press

SELECTED TITLES AVAILABLE IN THE SERIES

WRITING IMPERIAL HISTORIES
ed. Andrew S. Thompson

EMPIRE OF SCHOLARS
Tamson Pietsch

HISTORY, HERITAGE AND COLONIALISM
Kynan Gentry

COUNTRY HOUSES AND THE BRITISH EMPIRE
Stephanie Barczewski

THE RELIC STATE
Pamila Gupta

WE ARE NO LONGER IN FRANCE
Allison Drew

THE SUPPRESSION OF THE ATLANTIC SLAVE TRADE
ed. Robert Burroughs and Richard Huzzey

HEROIC IMPERIALISTS IN AFRICA
Berny Sèbe

Venomous encounters

SNAKES, VIVISECTION AND SCIENTIFIC MEDICINE IN COLONIAL AUSTRALIA

Peter Hobbins

MANCHESTER
UNIVERSITY PRESS

Published by MANCHESTER UNIVERSITY PRESS
ALTRINCHAM STREET, MANCHESTER M1 7JA

www.manchesteruniversitypress.co.uk

British Library Cataloguing-in-Publication Data
A catalogue record for this book is available from the British Library

Library of Congress Cataloging-in-Publication Data applied for

ISBN 978 1 5261 0144 0 hardback

First published 2017

Typeset by
Servis Filmsetting Ltd, Stockport, Cheshire
Printed in Great Britain by
TJ International Ltd, Padstow

For Solomon

CONTENTS

FIGURES

PREFACE

I am a repentant vivisector. This history is not, however, animated by an evangelical moralism. It emerged instead from a willingness to see and acknowledge animals as sentient agents, rather than mere apparatuses, in the processes and epistemology of science. As a budding pharmacologist I spent 1994 applying snake venoms to the dismembered remnants of laboratory animals. My disquiet at killing these creatures – and in the end my decision not to continue doing so – returned 15 years later when I commenced this analysis of nineteenth-century snakebite studies.

It proved possible to write individual animals into this history precisely because Victorian accounts foregrounded the presence and actions of experimental creatures in ways unthinkable to biomedical investigators after the mid-1920s. Acknowledging the extent of colonial snakebite studies also revealed a historiographic lacuna: the presumption that until the twentieth century, vivisection was confined almost exclusively to Western Europe. The corollary – a re-evaluation of the way that colonial science operated and circulated – drove the framing of this book as an animal-centred account. I hope that it at least captures something of the way in which each 'sacrificed' creature remained insistently individual.

ACKNOWLEDGEMENTS

I cannot begin to thank Alison Bashford enough for her mentorship and ever-insightful critique throughout the long research and writing process that resulted in this monograph. Her incisive intellect, strategic advice and collaborative ethos embody the spirit of scholarly collegiality at the heart of the university tradition. I also thank Claire Hooker for her encouraging words at every moment when my energies flagged and Ken Winkel for his enthusiastic support, including instigating the exhibition 'Venom: Fear, Fascination and Discovery' at the University of Melbourne Medical History Museum in 2013. Moreover, it would simply not have been possible to even contemplate this project without the unstinting love, understanding and forbearance of my wife, Rachel and my son, Will. Any errors within this work are, of course, mine alone.

Fellow scholars have been very generous with their advice and resources, particularly the late Peter Tyler and Barry Bryant. Jeanette Covacevich, Derek Dow, Martin Gibbs, Greg Haines, Ross Jones, Patricia Morison, John Pearn, John Shine and Michael Slouber all passed on sources, references, drafts and opinions. I particularly thank Charles Campbell and Sharon Wallace – my forerunners in exploring the history of Australian venom research – for the materials and enthusiasm they shared with me. The advice and encouragement provided by my doctoral thesis examiners – Michael Worboys, Harriet Ritvo and Libby Robin – have materially shaped the book before you and, indeed, made it possible. I also appreciate the perceptive challenges set for me by the reviewers of the draft manuscript.

The University of Sydney's Human–Animal Research Network provided an ongoing forum for discussing and thinking about animals in a scholarly context. Four friends stood out in changing the way that I conceived and created this book, and the way that I treat animals: Jodi Frawley, Hannah Forsyth, Miranda Johnson and Greg Murrie.

Numerous people and institutions ensured that the process of historical research remained an adventure with its own surprises and rewards. At the University of Sydney, I thank library staff Rena McGrogan, Jan Weaver and Bill Passlow; Jude Philp, Jan Brazier and Rob Blackburn at the Macleay Museum; Scott Lindsay and John Egerton in Veterinary Science; Nyree Morrison in the archives; and the office staff in Pharmacy who permitted me access to their uncatalogued historical collections. The Faculty of Arts and Social

Sciences has also been generous with research and travel grants. At the Melbourne University Medical History Museum, Ann Brothers, Susie Shields and Jackie Healy were all allies in making use of their unsurpassed resources. Stephen Due's Australian Medical Pioneers Index remained a constant resource for characterising early doctors. Barbara Morley and fellow descendants of George Halford have been helpful in locating family memorabilia, alongside Eulalie Brewster at the Inverloch Historical Society and Alan Humphries at the Thackray Museum. At the Yackandandah and District Historical Society, Susan Reynolds and Robyn Burns-Taylor helped fill out the beguiling stories of Augustus Mueller and Matthew Rome.

I also wish to acknowledge the archivists and special collections librarians at the Universities of Adelaide, Tasmania and Otago, plus Monash and James Cook Universities. The State Libraries of New South Wales and Victoria have, as always, proved invaluable. Liz Rouse at the Medical History Library of the Royal Australasian College of Physicians was an unstinting friend and enormous help. I am also grateful to the National Archives of Australia, Public Records Office of Victoria, State Records Office of Western Australia, State Records New South Wales, Archives Office of Tasmania and the Archives Office of New Zealand. I was particularly well looked after by Saribel Minero and Wayne Longmore at Museum Victoria, and Trish Egan at the Australian Museum.

Blessed with an editor as my life partner, I am ever aware of the prodigious thought and labour required to transform a mere manuscript into a published monograph. From the first the team at Manchester University Press have been personable and professional, reliable yet flexible. I sincerely thank them all for their roles in creating this contribution to an ongoing conversation about the past.

INTRODUCTION

From the day that Europeans first stepped ashore to occupy the Australian continent, they were never alone. From 1788, domesticated animals arrived alongside them, their numbers soon outstripping humans at every settlement. If colonists took comfort from the presence of these familiar beasts, they remained less certain of the indigenous creatures they encountered. Snakes, in particular, posed a quandary. Were they dangerous? What harm might they cause? And how could such *facts* be known?

This book argues that the practice of vivisection inextricably linked familiar animals and venomous snakes in colonial Australia. Over 1788–1914, imported beasts were both frequently observed and actively employed as victims of envenomation. While many instances were accidents, from 1840 onwards settlers increasingly orchestrated the transfer of venom from autochthonous serpents into living – and often unwilling – creatures. Even where it passed as entertainment, this process was primarily intended to find out something. Colonists hoped to determine the nature of snakes by discerning the action of their venom in other animals and – by extension – their own bodies (Figure 1).

This process – the empirical testing of animal toxins in sentient creatures – forms the analytical centre of *Venomous encounters*. Because such experiments employed living animals, I describe them as 'vivisection', although the meanings and nuances of that term shifted markedly over the nineteenth century.[1] While this practice is effectively absent from the historiography of colonial Australia, this book demonstrates that animal experiments to test venoms and putative antidotes were frequent, prominent and widespread across the antipodes prior to World War I. Yet if vivisection caused moral consternation in late Victorian Britain, in the Australian colonies such suffering went almost unremarked: studying snakebite intrinsically justified animal sacrifice. 'How could the action of snake poison ... be investigated', queried one Member of the Victorian Parliament in 1881, 'without cruelty to dogs?'[2] Thus the presumptive character of one group of animals shaped the ethical status of others.

Indeed vivisection, I contend, operated within a *colonial animal matrix*, a concept mapped out in Chapter 1. Each site of settlement generated a localised scaffold of animal hierarchies and equivalences, forging a series of commercial, moral and sentimental relationships

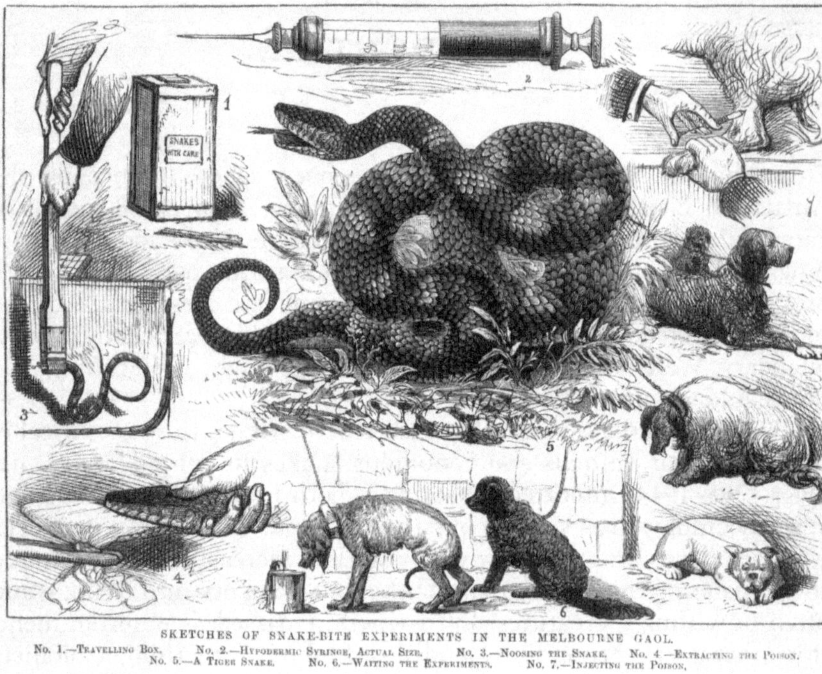

1 'Sketches of snakebite experiments in the Melbourne Gaol', *Australasian Sketcher with Pen and Pencil*, 17 February 1877.

between indigenous and imported creatures. As with a game of snakes and ladders, particular creatures might ascend, descend or move laterally through this matrix, reflecting dynamic perceptions of their worth. These evaluations constantly compared animals against each other, incorporating direct observations, environmental cues, intercolonial transactions and circulating narratives – including those legitimated via the coalescing structures of science or medicine.

The colonial stampede

Although non-Indigenous occupation of Australia commenced from 1788, the mid-1830s marked several critical turning points in antipodean colonisation. The first was a dramatic geographic, demographic and pastoral expansion, which saw both European settlers and their domesticated animals encroaching across vast new territories. After nearly 50 years of tightly corralled settlement in New South Wales and Van Diemen's Land, the demi-decade 1835–40 witnessed an upsurge in colonisation and galloping territorial encroachment, pushing deep inland and washing around the coastlines of Australia and New Zealand.

Accordingly, human and non-human encounters between invading and indigenous species escalated markedly. Yet as their purlieu expanded, settlers came to feel confident that the antipodes were bereft of threatening apex predators. Notwithstanding sharks and crocodiles, which rarely troubled whites until the twentieth century, in Australia the peak terrestrial carnivores were the 'native dog' or dingo, and the thylacine or 'Tasmanian tiger'. Neither species was dreaded in the manner of European wolves, American bears, Asiatic tigers or African lions.

The cultural and environmental place of such carnivores in subverting the colonial project has received considerable scholarly attention of late, emphasising both the agency of the creatures themselves and the complex geographies of encounter. Vividly recollecting her near death in the jaws of a crocodile, Australian ecofeminist Val Plumwood argues that for Europeans to become prey to non-human animals 'involves the forbidden mixing of these hyper-separated categories, the dissolution of the sacred–human into the profane–natural'.[3] The prospect – and spectacle – of claws and incisors violating white bodies undermines precarious presumptions of dominion while valorising the violent suppression of subaltern 'nature'.[4]

In contrast, what discomfited Australian colonists was not a fear of ending up inside a large predator, but the uncanny possibility that malign animal matter – venom – might contaminate their corporeal being.[5] I have elsewhere considered the transcolonial exchanges over poisonous spiders in New Zealand and Australia, as well as the atavistic implications of discovering that a 'primitive mammal' – the platypus – was also venomous.[6] But beyond the dreaded katipo spider, New Zealand proved peculiarly benign, as colonial boosters boasted: 'St. Patrick must have resided there before he discovered Ireland: there is not a snake or venomous reptile of any description whatever.'[7] If, as Pratik Chakrabarti emphasises, snakes 'formed an important part of the British imagination of Indian tropical wilderness', in the Australian colonies there was no question of their pre-eminence in the continent's ecology of dread (Figure 2).[8]

This obsession coincided with the third key development in antipodean human–animal relations: an upsurge in self-consciously local scientific activity. By the early 1840s Van Diemen's Land and New South Wales could boast relatively permanent learned societies, museums and periodicals purveying 'useful knowledge'. The subsequent circulation of intelligence within the antipodes provided a marked divergence from earlier scientific endeavours mediated largely via British authorities. The 1850s and beyond witnessed a gradual institutionalisation of science

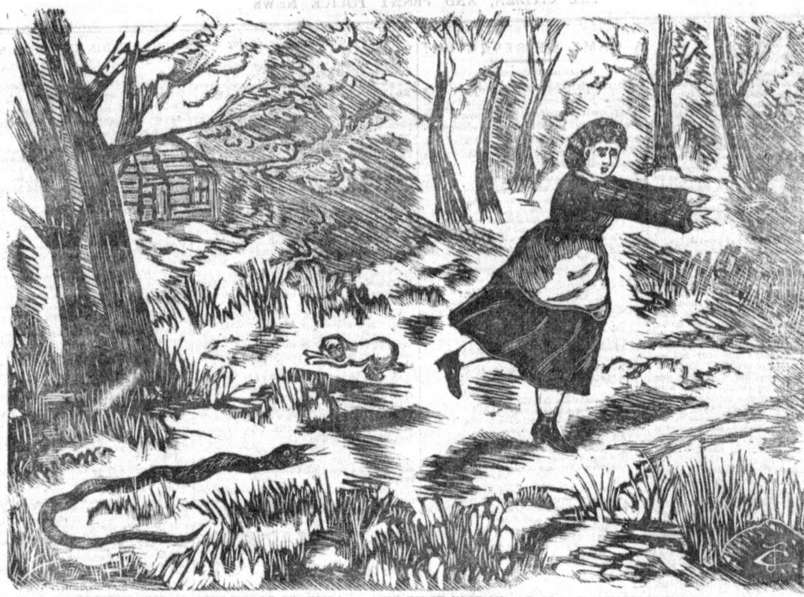

COMMENCEMENT OF THE SNAKE SEASON.——THE FIRST VICTIMS, AT COLAC AND WHITTLESEA.

2 'Commencement of the snake season. The first victims, at Colac and Whittlesea', *Police News*, 29 September 1877.

and medicine – in museums, mechanics' institutes, universities, hospitals, government departments and private enterprise – as a prominent but tenuous element of colonial culture.[9] As Chapters 2–6 elaborate, studies of snakes comprised an enduring if sporadic strand of inquiry that seamlessly spanned these local medical and scientific structures.

By the Federation of the Australian colonies in 1901, such ad hoc but rapidly professionalising pursuits were being palpably constrained by the limits of colonial infrastructure. Just as relations between publics and professions, science and government, medicine and experiment were transformed by World War I, so too were the ways in which animals were processed by twentieth-century schemas of zoology, veterinary science and biomedicine. As vivisection increasingly receded from the popular gaze through the *fin de siècle*, 1914 coincided with the end of a specifically colonial approach to knowing venomous serpents in Australia.

Speaking of animals

Much as they were often conflated, colonists consistently conceived snakes and their venoms as autonomous – and usually malevolent – agents. When 11-year-old John Howorth wilted and then died after the bite of a 'black snake' in 1804, 'a wound appeared upon the left arm, thro' which the noxious viper had poured the contaminating fluid'.[10] Foregrounding not just their presence but their potency in shaping colonial medical science is one of the primary missions of this book. Indeed, post-Enlightenment empiricism relied critically upon the testimony of non-humans, whether animals, microbes, instruments, spaces or the networks linking them. A Latourian focus on objects, performances, places and the translocation of agents is therefore central to how I delineate the material, literary and social technologies that – over the course of the nineteenth century – reduced sentient creatures to mere vessels for venom.[11]

Yet a key problem for actor–network theory lies in its propensity to flatten ethical gradations.[12] Important accounts of the rise of modern biomedicine also largely overlook the impact of instrumentation, quantification and atomisation upon its hecatombs of experimental animals.[13] But as Stephen Pemberton has demonstrated, not all animal subjects became objects: their innate character and behavioural choices can also impel a 'necessity to care'.[14] Furthermore, only recently have historians of colonial medical science – notably Pratik Chakrabarti – acknowledged that the ordering of animals entailed a conjoint operation of Imperial hierarchy and laboratory praxis.[15] If this 'ideological symbiosis' between empire and empiricism saw countless creatures 'sacrificed' for the instrumentalist ends of natural history or medicine,[16] Virginia DeJohn Anderson affirms that colonial animals also pursued their own ends, acting as both agents of European encroachment and mediators for Indigenous–invader relations.[17]

In elaborating the interactions between colonial practitioners and sentient creatures, *Venomous encounters* suggests that animals themselves structured scientific inquiry and its application to emergent debates in functional anatomy, germ theory, experimental physiology and immunology. In particular, it disrupts the smooth teleological narrative of biomedical modernity: that vivisection *necessarily* became a primary mode of medical progress.

An associated imperative is to comprehend the evolving but unstable nature of venom itself as an ontological agent. This formulation extends beyond Owsei Temkin's ontological conception of disease: the late nineteenth-century transition from remedying internal imbalances to perceiving discrete but stable external pathogens as the chief cause of illness.[18] Rather, I explore colonial characterisations of venom via the frame of objectivity championed by Lorraine Daston.[19] At stake was not merely an epistemology of knowing 'objective' facts, but the historical ontology of what could – or could not – be conceived to exist.[20] Comprehending the fundamental nature of venom – and its purposive relationship to the snake that expressed it – had cosmological consequences for Indigenous Australians and colonists alike.

Whilst the colonial animal matrix was predicated upon metonymic and emotive associations between humans and their animal familiars, this book does not attempt to historically reconstruct the interiority of snakes or other non-human creatures. In this decision I concur with Ludwig Wittgenstein's oft-cited aphorism, 'If a lion could talk, we could not understand him.'[21] Even when dealing with the charismatic species favoured by animal studies scholars, the sentience of non-human animals remains opaque to us. This does not mean, however, that we should not listen: the presence, intentions and actions of individual animals have meaning and consequence, even if they cannot adequately be translated into human terms.[22] Without attempting to rescue snakes from condescension, this book insists that denigrated, despised and dismissed creatures are also eminently worthy of consideration as historical actants.

Nevertheless, when venomous creatures encounter humans – or other animals – fear and suffering can commute in both directions. The results may be painful, distressing or lethal. In one sense, acknowledging this affective and embodied experience is important in understanding human animus towards snakes. Yet it was precisely the intersubjective identification with envenomed animals – above all, dogs – which reinforced the epistemological basis for vivisection in colonial Australia, even if it rarely translated into an ethical corollary.

Recognising the innate otherness of non-human animals also raises the vexed issues of essentialism, representation and naming. In writing this critical history of science and medicine, I have remained cautious of inscribing present-day conceptions onto historical circumstances. In part, this avoids simple linguistic pitfalls: the 'black snake' described by a British settler in 1820 may have borne little or no morphological relationship to the species presently characterised as the red-bellied black snake (*Pseudechis porphyriacus*). The animal may simply have been seen in poor light or, knowing that 'black snakes' were then considered deadly, the reporter may have employed this moniker to dramatise her account. The 'black snake' may simply have been a burnt stick. As such confusion over identification and nomenclature persists into the present, I have employed my protagonists' descriptions throughout the text without seeking to translate them taxonomically.

Conversely, I have been careful to reproduce names bestowed upon individual domestic animals. When his dog 'Duke' was bitten by a 'gray snake' in 1836, surveyor William Govett 'patted him, he got up, looked piteously in my face, and walked slowly after us' before staggering, collapsing and dying beside his horrified master.[23] Such accounts allow us to acknowledge each creature's unique identity, while serving as an analytical device for tracing shifting historical relations of ownership, sentimental attachment and moral consideration.[24]

The historical veracity of reported bites and subsequent symptomatology is notoriously difficult to ascertain. Thus individual case reports and colonial statistics on envenomation must be interpreted with extreme caution. Even apparently neutral descriptors such as 'envenomation' may carry anachronistic biomedical implications inappropriate or meaningless, for instance, to Indigenous cosmologies. Furthermore, animals are individuals, not archetypes. Characters observed in the present day – from the 'tameness' of an escaped cow to the potency of a serpent's venom – can and do change over individual lifetimes, let alone two centuries. I have therefore sought not to impose contemporary medical or toxinological data onto historical accounts, nor to attempt retrospective diagnoses. Rather, I have tried to integrate consideration of the actors involved, depicting how historical conjunctions – of animals, toxins, humans, equipment, spaces and discourses – continuously renegotiated the place of venomous creatures in the colonial animal matrix.

Structure and analytical threads

This book's primary argument is that over 1840–1914, vivisection proved both divisive and decisive in colonial Australia, dramatically changing local perceptions of venomous snakes and their toxins. These shifts occurred within the larger schema of a colonial animal matrix, which structured the moral, sentimental and commercial worth of animals in relation to other creatures.

Global scholarship on the messy menageries of colonialism increasingly affirms that, from the Transvaal to Tasmania, animals 'occupied material and symbolic spaces, helping to buttress the shifting socio-political orders and looming large in rituals of social differentiation'.[25] Each of the scattered settlements typifying the colonial antipodes comprised an unstable conjunction of people, animals, environments, technologies and circumstances, providing a rich source for animal-focused histories.[26] As detailed in Chapter 1, abrupt shifts in economic, ethical or affective valuations of animals threw into relief prevailing attitudes and practices. This chapter establishes the concept of the colonial animal matrix, elaborating how white settlers related both to the domestic species that landed alongside them and the autochthonous animals they encountered up to 1840. Even as these localised hierarchies multiplied, by 1820 the settlers had established a consistent folkbiology for Australian serpents, based largely upon observing accidental snakebites in their valuable imported domesticates.

Chapter 2 characterises lay expertise in regard to snakebite and remedies, especially over 1840–80. Outlining European folklore and Aboriginal practices, I argue that by the early 1850s, plebeian expertise had established vivisection as the prime means of knowing venomous animals in Australia. In particular, snake charmers and antidote spruikers widely performed 'experiments' which involved the envenomation – and usually the suffering and death – of familiar domestic animals. Because these vivisections so frequently engaged general audiences, more was at stake than merely the evidence tendered. The very nature of proof itself was under negotiation. Indeed, into the 1870s lay practitioners – and the publics who attended their shows – embraced the epistemology of vivisection far more readily than doctors or naturalists. These professionals were, in fact, impelled to adopt animal experimentation largely because of its plebeian popularity.

Historians have frequently elaborated the impact of Australia's unique fauna upon the European imagination, from black swans to kangaroos.[27] Rarely explored, however, is the way in which animal poisons were perceived or investigated. Chapter 3 argues that, from 1840, local scientific and medical cultures shifted away from anatomical description and clinical testimony in determining which indigenous beasts were dangerous. By comparing the characterisation of local snakes with the potential emergence of rabies as a 'venomous' disease, I contend that instruments and living experiments became necessary to establish *objective* medical facts in the antipodes. As these exchanges coincided with the emergence of germ theories of disease, venom provided both an enigma and an exemplar of an ontological agent of disease. Yet neither microscopy nor vivisection could firmly establish its status as a living or dead entity, especially when Australian observations were nullified by international interlocutors.

In transitioning from a deferential tradition favouring scriptural, classical or clinical authority, colonial doctors and scientists rarely embraced positivism in a rigorous Comtean sense. Spanning the critical decade of 1868 to 1876, Chapter 4 details how snakebite treatment and vivisection were central to a profuse and acrimonious medical debate across British Australia and India. At stake were competing discourses and practices of medical authority, encompassing clinical testimony, observations in animals and public participation. Even as they became tools for experiment, however, domesticated creatures emerged as patients for Australian snakebite remedies. As this chapter demonstrates, the moral devaluation of experimental animals did not silence their ability to 'speak' as subjects. Nevertheless, this decade proved decisive for the heuristics of colonial medicine. By the time that Britain legislatively regulated vivisection in mid-1876, animal experimentation had independently become de rigueur for colonial investigations of envenomation and remedies.

Centred on the 1880s, Chapter 5 complicates the moral and epistemological status of animal experimentation. In 1881 the colony of Victoria became the second legislature worldwide to formally regulate vivisection, yet both the spirit and enforcement of this law were honoured mainly in the breach. This statute arose, I argue, to protect human investigators rather than their animal subjects. Indeed, seeking an effective remedy for snakebite was considered sufficient reason to lessen moral consideration for all animals involved in such experiments. Through the emergence of a novel injected remedy – subcutaneous strychnine – this chapter furthermore affirms that well into the 1890s there was no certitude that vivisection would succeed clinical experience as the fundamental epistemology underscoring colonial medical practice.

Concluding with the outbreak of World War I, Chapter 6 reprises the authority claims outlined in Chapter 4. Contrasting Australia with India and French Indo-China, clinical experience appeared largely to trump vivisectional data for much of the 1890s. Yet when a 'universal' antivenene appeared – predicated upon the new science of immunology – its efficacy was concomitantly discredited by the novel technologies of experimental medicine. In particular, animal studies suggested that because venoms were complex biochemical mixtures, geographically specific antivenenes would be required to counter the venom of each local species. Australia concurrently became an independent nation, whose citizens increasingly valued their native fauna. For snakes, however, this transformation represented a hollow victory. As venom came to be seen as a potent autonomous agent, snakes were correspondingly drained of the awe they had once commanded.

For settlers in the Australian colonies, public vivisections to study envenomation and antidotes established standards of proof and authority which were followed, rather than led, by learned professionals. By tracing the tools, techniques and arguments through which venomous animals and their toxins were characterised, this book offers a new perspective not only on science and medicine in the colonial antipodes, but of their wider impact upon animals in the nineteenth-century world.

Notes

1 The foundational text is Richard D. French, *Antivivisection and Medical Science in Victorian Society* (Princeton: Princeton University Press, 1975). See also Andreas-Holger Maehle and Ulrich Tröhler, 'Animal experimentation from antiquity to the end of the eighteenth century: attitudes and arguments', in Nicolaas Rupke (ed.), *Vivisection in Historical Perspective* (London: Croom Helm, 1987), pp. 30–9; Anita Guerrini, *Experimenting with Humans and Animals: From Galen to Animal Rights* (Baltimore: Johns Hopkins University Press, 2003), pp. 61–74.

2 *Victoria. Parliamentary Debates. Session 1881. Legislative Council and Legislative Assembly* (Melbourne: John Ferres, 1882), p. 344.

3 Val Plumwood, 'Human vulnerability and the experience of being prey', *Quadrant,* 39:3 (1995), p. 34.

4 For example, Heather Schell, 'Tiger tales', in Deborah Denenholz Morse and Martin A. Danahay (eds), *Victorian Animal Dreams: Representations of Animals in Victorian Literature and Culture* (Aldershot: Ashgate, 2007), pp. 230–48; Mark V. Barrow Jr, 'The alligator's allure: changing perceptions of a charismatic carnivore', in Dorothee Brantz, ed., *Beastly Natures: Animals, Humans, and the Study of History* (Charlottesville: University of Virginia Press, 2010), pp. 127–53; Chris Wilbert, 'What is doing the killing? animal attacks, man-eaters, and shifting boundaries and flows of human–animal relations', in The Animal Studies Group (eds), *Killing Animals* (Urbana: University of Illinois Press, 2006), pp. 30–49.

5 This sense of 'uncanny' owes a debt to Julia Kristeva; see James Hatley, 'Where the beaver gnaw: predatory space in the urban landscape', in Gary Backhaus and John Murungi (eds), *Transformations of Urban and Suburban Landscapes: Perspectives from Philosophy, Geography, and Architecture* (Lanham: Lexington Books, 2002), pp. 39–40.

6 Peter Hobbins, 'Invasion ontologies: venom, visibility and the imagined histories of arthropods', in Jodi Frawley and Iain McCalman (eds), *Rethinking Invasion Ecologies from the Environmental Humanities* (Oxford: Routledge, 2014), pp. 181–95; Peter Hobbins, 'A spur to atavism: placing platypus poison', *Journal of the History of Biology* (2015), pp. 499–537.

7 Charles Hursthouse, *New Zealand, or Zealandia, the Britain of the South,* vol. I (London: Edward Stanford, 1857), pp. 117–18.

8 Pratik Chakrabarti, *Bacteriology in British India: Laboratory Medicine and the Tropics* (Rochester: University of Rochester Press, 2012), p. 116.

9 See Bryan Gandevia and Ann Tovell, 'The first Australian medical libraries', *Medical Journal of Australia,* 2 (1964), pp. 314–20; Colin Finney, *Paradise Revealed: Natural History in Nineteenth-Century Australia* (Melbourne: Museum of Victoria, 1993), pp. 1–62.

10 'Sydney', *Sydney Gazette and New South Wales Advertiser* (21 October 1804), p. 3.

11 Bruno Latour, *The Pasteurization of France,* trans. Alan Sheridan and John Law (Cambridge, Mass.: Harvard University Press, 1988), pp. 22–39; David N. Livingstone, *Putting Science in its Place: Geographies of Scientific Knowledge* (Chicago: University of Chicago Press, 2003), pp. 141–85; Steven Shapin and Simon Schaffer, *Leviathan and the Air Pump: Hobbes, Boyle, and the Experimental Life* (Princeton: Princeton University Press, 2011), pp. 22–40.

12 Tim Ingold, 'When ANT meets SPIDER: social theory for arthropods', in Carl Knappett and Lambros Malafouris (eds), *Material Agency: Towards a Non-Anthropocentric Approach* (New York: Springer, 2008), pp. 209–15.

13 For instance, Michael Worboys, *Spreading Germs: Disease Theories and Medical Practice in Britain, 1865–1900* (Cambridge: Cambridge University Press, 2000); W.F. Bynum, 'The rise of science in medicine, 1850–1913', in W.F. Bynum *et al.* (eds), *The Western Medical Tradition, 1800 to 2000* (Cambridge: Cambridge University Press, 2006), pp. 103–239.

14 Stephen Pemberton, 'Canine technologies, model patients: the historical produc-

tion of hemophiliac dogs in American biomedicine', in Susan Schrepfer and Philip Scranton (eds), *Industrializing Organisms: Introducing Evolutionary History* (New York: Routledge, 2004), pp. 202–5. See also Lynda Birke, *Feminism, Animals and Science: The Naming of the Shrew* (Buckingham: Open University Press, 1994), pp. 43–7.

15 Pratik Chakrabarti, 'Beasts of burden: animals and laboratory research in colonial India', *History of Science*, 48:2 (2010), pp. 125–51.

16 Richard Drayton, 'Science, medicine, and the British Empire', in Robin W. Winks and Alaine Low (eds), *The Oxford History of the British Empire* (Oxford: Oxford University Press, 1999), p. 264.

17 Virginia DeJohn Anderson, *Creatures of Empire: How Domestic Animals Transformed Early America* (Oxford: Oxford University Press, 2004), pp. 160–71, 211–16.

18 Owsei Temkin, 'The scientific approach to disease: specific entity and individual sickness', in A.C. Crombie (ed.), *Scientific Change: Historical Studies in the Intellectual, Social, and Technical Conditions for Scientific Discovery and Technical Invention, from Antiquity to the Present* (London: Heinemann, 1963), pp. 629–47.

19 Lorraine Daston and Peter Galison, *Objectivity* (New York: Zone Books, 2007), pp. 19–27.

20 Ian Hacking, *Historical Ontology* (Cambridge, Mass.: Harvard University Press, 2002), pp. 1–26.

21 Ludwig Wittgenstein, *Philosophical Investigations*, 2nd edn, trans. G.E.N. Anscombe (Oxford: Basil Blackwell, 1963), p. 223e. See also Cary Wolfe, 'In the shadow of Wittgenstein's lion: language, ethics, and the question of the animal', in Cary Wolfe (ed.), *Zoontologies: The Question of the Animal* (Minneapolis: University of Minnesota Press, 2003), pp. 1–57.

22 Key texts include Jacques Derrida, 'The animal that therefore I am (more to follow)', trans. David Willis, *Critical Inquiry*, 28 (2002), pp. 369–418; Donna Haraway, *The Companion Species Manifesto: Dogs, People, and Significant Otherness* (Chicago: Prickly Paradigm, 2003), pp. 3–25; Akira Mizuta Lipitt, *Electric Animal: Toward a Rhetoric of Wildlife* (Minneapolis: University of Minnesota Press, 2008), pp. 1–25.

23 State Library of New South Wales, Sydney, A 330, Notes and sketches taken during a surveying Expedition in N. South Wales and Blue Mountains Road by William Govett on staff of Major Mitchell, Surveyor General of New South Wales, William Romaine Govett, 1830–1835, p. 11.

24 Harriet Ritvo, 'Our animal cousins', *differences: A Journal of Feminist Cultural Studies*, 15:1 (2004), pp. 48–68.

25 Sandra Swart, *Riding High: Horses, Humans and History in South Africa* (Johannesburg: Witwatersrand University Press, 2010), p. 2.

26 See for instance Robert Kenny, *The Lamb Enters the Dreaming: Nathanael Pepper & the Ruptured World* (Melbourne: Scribe, 2007), pp. 168–76.

27 Examples include Penny Olsen, *Upside Down World: Early European Impressions of Australia's Curious Animals* (Canberra: National Library of Australia, 2010), pp. 2–5; Danielle Clode, 'From molluscs to monkeys: Darwin and early Australian biology', in Jeanette Hoorn (ed.), *Reframing Darwin: Evolution and the Arts in Australia* (South Carlton: Melbourne University Press, 2009), pp. 14–19.

CHAPTER ONE

Serpents and settlers: the colonial animal matrix, 1788–1840

In 1836, on the cusp of Queen Victoria's coronation, retired colonial surveyor William Govett reassured British readers that 'Venomous snakes are now but rarely seen in England, and all danger from them nearly at an end.' Serpents in New South Wales, however, were another matter. Although small and timid, 'they make up for that deficiency by the deadly nature of their venom'.[1] Concurrently, former convict Richard Bowler scrawled from Van Diemen's Land,

> there his but few wild animals and none injurious there his the tiger she will destroy sheep but will run away from any person there his the opposum kangaroo rat wharmbat dog devils the snake his very venemous here where the bite if the piece is not cut instantly it is almost sure death at sundown the scorpion his venemous but not like the snake.[2]

Whatever their relative stations and literary merits, these colonial correspondents clearly shared a truth borne out by history – natural history to be exact.

Commencing in 1788 – and thus coinciding with the release of Gilbert White's *The Natural History of Selborne* – by 1840 British colonisation of Australia had spanned the heyday of natural history. Most studies of this historical convergence foreground collecting. The accumulation of specimens, descriptions and information is central to narratives of early antipodean science and its problematic relationship with patrons, audiences and institutions in Europe.[3] Few scholars, however, have detailed the generation, circulation or application of natural knowledge *within* the Australasian colonies before 1840.

Indeed, historians remain divided as to when a scientific culture was truly established in the antipodes. Learned societies first arose in New South Wales from 1820, as did local libraries and periodicals for disseminating 'useful knowledge'. By 1844, Van Diemen's Land became the first location beyond Britain to found a Royal Society.[4] Yet until the mid-1850s, antipodean doctors relied upon local newspapers and European journals for professional exchange. Scientific infrastructure remained spartan until the gold rushes reshaped colonial fortunes from 1851.

This chapter argues, however, that a local epistemology of natural history developed beyond such institutional forms. Specifically, by 1820 colonists had established a robust schema for determining which indigenous snakes were dangerous. In the historiography – and in many nineteenth-century sources – this process appears unproblematic: all that was required to render a snake 'venomous' was the presence of a naturalist. In 1821 *The Australian Magazine* – the first antipodean periodical to entertain scientific conceits – featured an article on snakes within its inaugural volume.[5] This pattern was perpetuated by almost every scientific, natural history and medical and pharmacy journal published in Australia before World War I.

But such information was never simply observed: it was *generated*. Human snakebite cases certainly contributed, but equally important were the domestic animals which arrived alongside the colonists. Observing the effects of poisons in living creatures was important to lay understanding of the natural world.

Furthermore, while snakebites before 1840 were usually considered 'accidents', thereafter passive experience turned increasingly to active experiment – specifically, vivisection. Experiments in animals were frequently conducted not by authoritative figures, but by plebeian investigators. From the 1860s, medical and scientific practitioners studying snakebite also gravitated toward vivisection, yet the resultant 'scientific medicine' remained divisive until 1914.

The fading bestiary tradition

As the medieval era waned, the place of animals in western culture was informed by quotidian contact, allegorical nuance and above all by biblical authority.[6] Yet if God created creatures to serve the ends of man, Genesis 3:14 affirmed that God cursed the serpent 'above all cattle, and above every beast of the field'. Dwelling suspiciously close to the underworld, snakes were loathed in Leviticus 11:29 as the unclean 'creeping things that creep along the earth'.[7] As Esther Cohen remarks, they also served alongside bears and lions as earthly reminders of God's terrifying power.[8] This exegetical tradition endured into the era of colonial encounters with threatening beasts, from American alligators to Sumatran tigers.

Although rarely overlapping with modern conceptions of zoonoses, vectors or venom, many 'brutes' were attributed with the ability to cause – or cure – illness. Early modern bestiaries were typified by an indiscriminate intermingling – of authority and hearsay, 'zoology' and medicine, pragmatism and morality.[9] In his pivotal *The Historie of Serpents* (1608), English pastor Edward Topsell enumerated all 65 known 'venemous beasts', from adders to elephants, scorpions to dragons. People were 'poysoned, envenomed, or bitten', he explained, because these creatures were motivated by a 'deepe hatred to mankind'.[10]

Victims, however, were never just human. Topsell's contemporaries held serpents and dragons responsible for 'the great annoyance and divers slaughters both of Men and Cattell, by [their] strong & violent poyson'.[11] His medical advice likewise layered animal associations: applying a chicken's fundament to a snakebite assuaged symptoms because, 'beeing of a very hot nature and complexion, [it will] easilie concoct and digest notable poyson'.[12]

What united such measures was Topsell's ontology of poisons: material agents which operated autonomously inside 'all such persons as be wounded by venomous creatures'. If each noxious beast produced specific poisonous effects, his primary remedy was a ligature above the bite to ensure 'that the poyson may not too easily convey itself, and penetrate into the more noble and principall parts, as the hart, liver or braine'. This tourniquet was to be followed by scarification, excision, amputation or cauterisation of the bite site to destroy or expel the venom. Sucking or attaching 'attractives' to the bite site, such as half a dove or the fresh entrails of a goat, would 'draw out the poyson and mittigate paine'.[13]

Yet the toxic *nature* of venom was an elusive entity. Throughout the middle ages, as Kathleen Walker-Meikle observes, 'nearly all medical authors followed Avicenna in claiming that it was a "hot" poison', but rarely endowed it with supernatural potency.[14] Even as they banished basilisks to the outlands of credulity (Figure 3), European writers detailed how animal poisons were communicated not merely through bites or stings, but in saliva, breath, blood, urine or a 'horrid look'.[15] As the tentacles of English colonialism embraced the globe, hot climates were accused of enhancing the aggressiveness of snakes and the potency of their poison. It proved an enduring trope.

Malevolent intentions: indignant serpents and enraged spirits

By the Restoration, European anatomists had effectively overthrown the Galenic dogma that venom originated in bile. Rather, they reasoned, it was a form of saliva generated in vesicles behind the serpent's fangs.[16] But did noxiousness lie within the venom itself, or in the

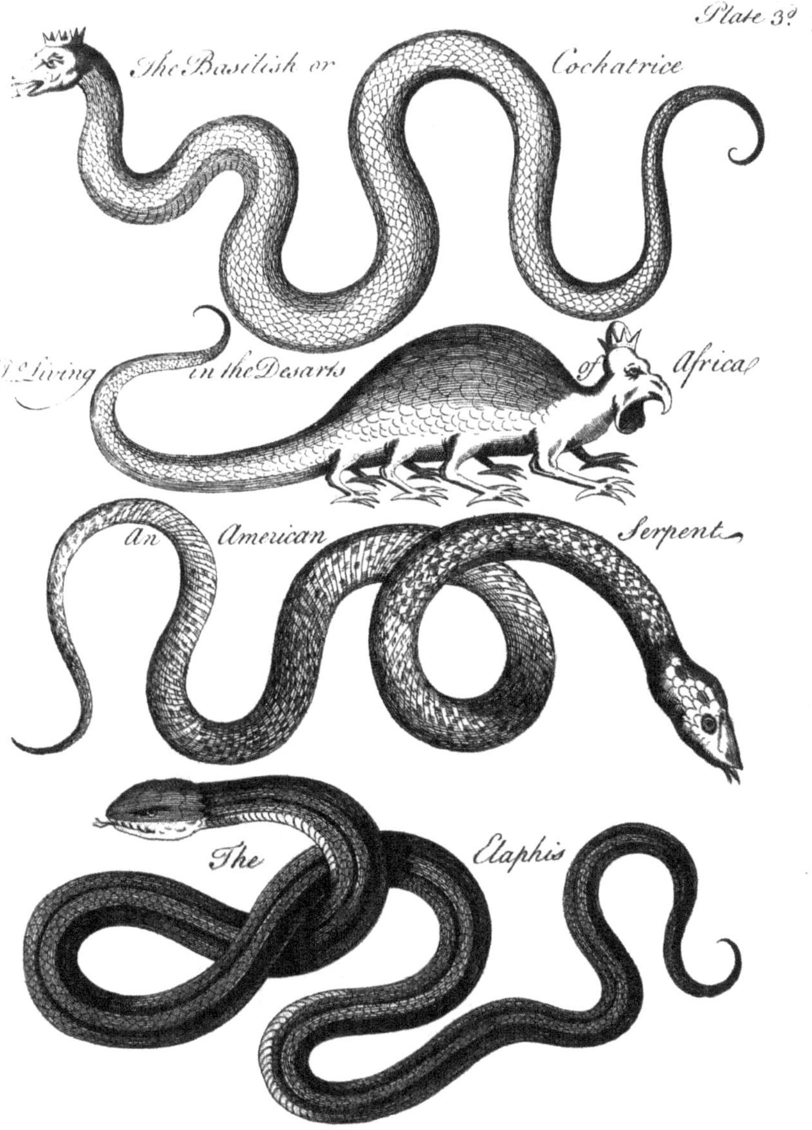

3 Charles Owen, *An Essay towards a Natural History of Serpents* (London: Charles Owen, 1742).

serpent's malevolent intentions? Furthermore, should experimental philosophy supplement classical and clinical authority, or supplant it?

In 1670, French apothecary Moyse Charas argued that new knowledge of vipers could arise only via dissections and 'Experiments tried of their biting, upon divers Animals'. Amongst his pigeons, fowls, cats and dogs was a hound which struggled vigorously but vainly to avoid a fatal bite forced upon his tongue. 'This last Experiment gave us great satisfaction', Charas boasted, 'shewing us, that the poyson goes not directly to the noble parts ... but that 'tis chiefly the bloud it works upon'.[17] Claiming that 'the cause of the Venom is to be imputed to the Spirits enraged, and not to any other thing or parts in the Vipers body', he found an ally in British physician Henry Stubbe who agreed that 'the *venome* of the Animal proceeds from its *indignation*'.[18]

Concurring on the value of investigative experiences, Florentine physician-naturalist Francesco Redi dismissed Charas's influential ontology. In his 1664 monograph on their 'juice', Redi reported killing hundreds of vipers for their venom, introducing it into doves, pigeons, chickens, ducks, turtles, rabbits, lambs and dogs.[19] As both the living embodiment of the antidote–poison paradox and the subject of enduring philosophical inquiry, suggests Jay Tribby, vipers provided 'a perfect object for the profit and delight of any civil interlocutor in the seventeenth century'.[20]

Indeed, Redi's studies embodied a new modus for natural philosophy: no longer merely discursive, interventions were also performative. Staging vivisections before crowds of witnesses because 'while humans might be guilty of fraud or deception, animals would not', he demonstrated that venom remained potent even weeks after the serpent was killed.[21] Yet Redi's recourse to vivisection only exacerbated medical discord.[22] Although often cited, his experiences rarely overturned wider cultural associations between the anger of a biting animal and the potency of its venom. Indeed, into the nineteenth century, medical treatises commonly conflated venomous snakes and rabid dogs as 'enraged animals', a trope regularly recapitulated in colonial contexts – especially India.[23]

Moreover, in the Anglophone world, Redi's vivisections and opinions remained secondary to those of Richard Mead. Later appointed physician to George II, Mead established his reputation in 1702 with *A Mechanical Account of Poisons*, regularly revised and plagiarised throughout the ensuing century. Tormenting vipers, Mead forced them upon dogs, cats and pigeons, or used decapitated heads and hollow steel needles to inoculate venom into luckless brutes. Asserting that the universal effect of poisons was that 'the animal œconomy is all disturbed ... [and] the first bad impression is made upon the animal spirits', he defined venoms as a 'liquor ... which infects the fluid of the nerves, and by this means inflames the membranes [so that] a swelling arises, sometimes to a degree of mortification, which spreads to the neighbouring parts'.[24]

By the early eighteenth century, physicians wavered between vital and chemical explanations of venom, representing the emergence of both chemistry and Paracelsian theory. Contending that discrete maladies were manifestations of uniform underlying causes, Paracelsus urged physicians to eschew symptomatic remedies for 'specifics' targeting this aetiology. Poisons, he argued, were not innately noxious; they merely awaited Man's ingenuity to discern their divinely ordained virtues.[25]

Venom, viruses and prolific matter

While discord reigned, all authors agreed that a discrete substance passed from serpent to victim. In 1736, English physician Daniel Turner specified that venom arose in animals from 'such a peculiar Disorder as transforms them from their mild and benign Nature, to one so very malignant, that the whole *Systasis* of the corporeal Soul is carry'd into a Sort of Fury, Outrage or Madness'.[26] Thus, ventured physician Richard Brookes in *The General Practice of Physic*, the 'Venom of Animals, whether in a Rage or Madness, communicates an Infection not only by the *Saliva*, *Milk*, and *Lympha*, but by the *Semen*, whence Women have received the Contagion from their Husbands'.[27]

Indeed, it was an Enlightenment refrain that venom 'infected' its recipient, commonly associating the poison of serpents with the agents of fever and contagion. The most frequent conjunction was snakebite and rabies, considered communicable via the bite of an 'enraged' canine. But as Stanford Wolsterstan asserted in his 1692 tract on humoral medicine, 'there is nothing as I have (yet) observed, doth more exactly represent, or express the Nature of the Plague unto us ... than the first biteings of a strong Viper'.[28] Encouraging snakes to bite dogs, he asserted that the potency of venom resided not in the serpent's 'spirit', but its inanimate fluid.

By the 1760s a new term – 'virus' – described an active particle which could multiply or otherwise exert malign influence beyond its initial nidus. Following a viper bite, 'a train of particular symptoms ... seem to be caused by the *stimuli* or sharp pungent saline *spiculæ* of the virus', observed surgeon Peter Shaw in 1753.[29] 'How subtle, how penetrating, how divisible, must the component Particles of this little Speck of Venom be!' enthused microscopist Henry Baker in 1769.[30]

Did this aetiological agent, therefore, possess its own vital properties? Georges-Louis Buffon, by far the most influential natural historian of the late eighteenth century, considered spiculae not salts – as Mead proposed – but 'organic particles in an extremely active state'.[31] They were, he argued in 1780, variants of the motile 'prolific matter' residing in seminal fluid, putrefying wounds, decomposing vegetables, and on the teeth of vipers and mad dogs. Assuming all manner of living forms, these pluripotent particles pursued a productive existence – sometimes benign, often malign – completely distinct from the intentions of the host animal.

'A Race hateful to us': the rightful place of snakes

By 1788, European management of snakebite had long consisted of two intertwined strands: physical arrest of the movement of venom and its neutralisation by antidotes. The former, as Topsell outlined in 1608, might comprise cautery, cutting or sucking the bitten part to bleed out the poison, or tying a ligature above the wound. Medical remedies – including plasters, poultices, unguents and draughts – were prescribed according to established authority, the idiosyncrasies of the patient and the whim of the physician.

Theriac was a special case. As a universal antidote intended to fortify the body against all poisons by introducing small doses of them, viper flesh remained critical amongst its scores of ingredients.[32] By the Restoration, however, this extraordinarily complex and somewhat mystical panacea was fading before simpler Paracelsian therapeutics, seeking to counteract venom just as acid neutralised alkali. The effectiveness of such specifics was established not merely in human patients; surgeon James Handley valued 'above all, the *Auxungia Viperarum* [viper fat], by which it is thought that the *Viper Catchers* cure themselves, and Dogs when bitten'.[33]

In colonial contexts, especially India, microscopic study, chemical analysis and Paracelsian theory often stood in awkward conjunction with localised knowledges of serpents and snakebite antidotes. Epistemologies which incorporated indigenous recipes and cosmologies, details Pratik Chakrabarti, 'had their distinct orientations in different locales, and during their transmission many of the insights gained, along with the items and materials of science, were eroded'.[34] For instance, vernacular 'Tanjore pills' were almost ubiquitously trusted by Indians and European colonists for the bites of snakes and mad dogs. At first embraced, then dismissed following British botanical and vivisectional analysis in the 1780s, they enjoyed an extended local afterlife.

Yet western concern over 'poisonous' Indian remedies endured, particularly when their names, constituents and properties proved unstable across regions, merchants and practitioners.[35] This ontological incommensurability was typified by the multiple incarnations and evaluations of theriac, tiryaq faruq and treeak farook across Eurasia which, Guy Attewell elaborates, made it 'impossible to disaggregate medicinal effect, materiality and its socially embedded powers'.[36]

Reason, moreover, remained but one authority for knowing the natural world. Exegetical tracts of natural theology ascribed meaning and morals to the fruits of creation. 'The very Serpents, though a Race hateful to us, have their uses', allowed the Lord Archbishop of Dublin in 1732, for 'they may serve to gather Poison out of the Earth'.[37] In his prodigious *Essay Towards a Natural History of Serpents* of 1742, Lancashire minister Charles Owen remarked, 'if Serpents, and other venemous Creatures, are hurtful to us, 'tis only by Accident'.[38] Not all agreed with such mild cosmologies. In 1777 the plagiarised *Beauties of Natural History* asserted that from the day the serpent tempted Adam, 'the early malignity of this dreadful race [created] the most fatal and lasting mischief ... our natural antipathy seems natural and permanent'.[39]

But if clerics were comforted by the relative innocuousness of British serpents, a new challenge arose not from exegesis, but via colonial expansion. Feared from the 1660s, in the eighteenth century the American rattlesnake was considered the deadliest serpent on Earth. In particular, a series of experiments critical to British philosophical opinion was communicated from South Carolina to the Royal Society in 1727. Ship's captain Fayer Hall forced a rattlesnake to bite a series of dogs, a cat, hen, bull-frog, another snake and then itself. The results, he asserted, affirmed that rattlesnake venom was almost universally deadly. Hall would gladly have killed more animals to satisfy his curiosity but, he complained, 'Dogs and Cats were not to be had; for the good Women, whose Dogs had been killed, exclaimed so much, that I durst not meddle with one afterwards'.[40]

The impact of such colonial experiences was profound. Hearing Hall's assertion that a rattlesnake bite killed a dog in a quarter of a minute, Richard Mead changed his fundamental conception of poisons. As its venom was 'more quick and deadly' than any known poison, such rapidity could not be explained by circulation through the blood.[41] Rather, presumed Mead, the nerves must be the conduit through which poisons assailed the animal spirits. While many contemporaries agreed, others insisted that the rattlesnake's temperament was equally important, proving dangerous only when provoked.

While such folkbiological knowledge of 'dangerous' animals shaped the quotidian names and practices employed by settlers on the ground, it also percolated into the semiotic systems that characterised colonial species and spaces.[42] 'As one of the most dangerous animals of India and Africa, the crocodile literally stood in the way of colonial settlement', Mary Leighton and Lisa Surridge insist. Functioning 'as the quintessential sign of alterity ... the reptile came to represent the fear of colonial treachery, uprising, or sneak attack'.[43] Eighteenth-century cartographers literally mapped crocodilians onto the landscape of south-eastern North America, a cartouche bespeaking both menacing otherness and an impediment to European encroachment.[44] From wolves to lions, as Harriet Ritvo asserts, 'British settlers and colonizers set themselves parallel physical and metaphorical challenges, conflating the elimination of dangerous animals with the imposition of political and military order.'[45]

If this animal world did not escape the global realignment of colonial possessions after the Seven Years' War, snakes continued to bite back. By 1775, vicar Samuel Ward asserted in *A Modern System of Natural History* that the Indian '*cobra di capello*, or *hooded serpent*, inflicts the most deadly and incurable wounds ... a speedy death being the certain consequence of their bite'.[46] In 1793 none other than Buffon pontificated that 'when the person is bit by the cobra di capello, he dies in an hour, his whole frame being dissolved into a putrid mass of corruption'.[47] 'Nothing', observed Oliver Goldsmith in *An History of the Earth, and Animated Nature* (1779), 'can more justly excite our wonder than that so small a quantity of venom should produce such powerful and deadly effects.'[48]

While natural histories continued to catalogue winged serpents through to the end of the eighteenth century, by 1780 the era of credulous bestiaries was closing. With observation trumping revelation, Goldsmith explained that venomous serpents could be known by the possession of a pair of hollow fangs in their upper jaws. If his volumes marked a transition from the realm of Creation to the works of Nature, they also cautioned against colonial hubris in presuming that dominion implied domination. 'Mankind have driven the lion, the tiger and the wolf from their vicinity, but the snake and the viper still defy their power, and frequently punish their insolence', he cautioned. 'Nature seems to have placed them as centinels [*sic*] to deter mankind from spreading too widely.'[49]

Evident marks and characters

Whether snakes stood sentinel against the invasion of Australia was not immediately apparent. That serpents inhabited the southern landmass – or at least its waters – had been known in Britain since William Dampier's 1703 account of New Holland. Nevertheless, Britons arriving to colonise Port Jackson in 1788 were nonchalant. 'The species of Serpents are much less easily ascertained that those of most other animals', complained Surgeon-General John White in his

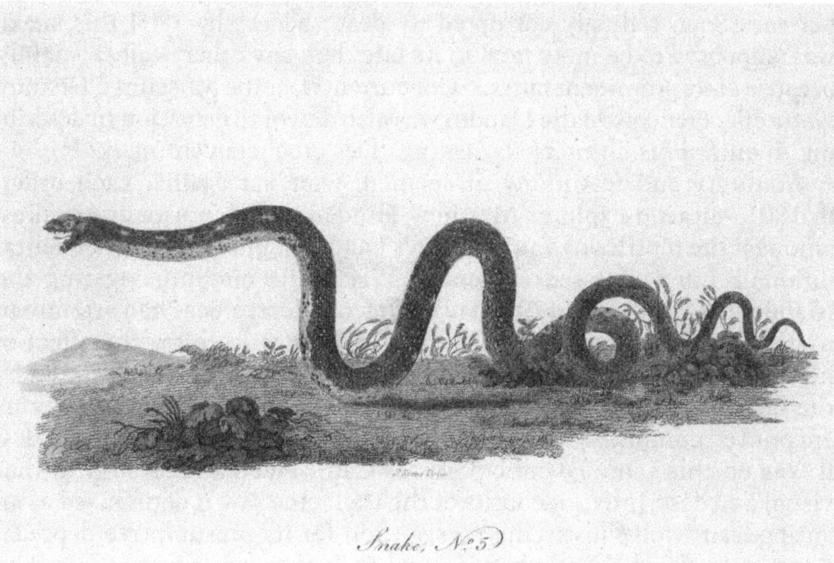

4 Sarah Stone, 'Snake, No. 5', in John White, *Journal of a Voyage to New South Wales* (London: I. Debrett, 1789).

1790 account of the new settlement. Happily, none appeared 'to be of a poisonous nature' (Figure 4).[50]

Indeed, no warning accompanied the European debut of the 'crimson-sided snake' in George Shaw's *Zoology of New Holland* (1794). This imputed benignity seems curious, given the longevity of the Paracelsian doctrine of signatures, a providentialist theology which asserted that 'the most noxious animals have evident marks and characters, by which their dangerous properties are easily known'.[51] Despite its prominent red belly, Shaw deemed *Coluber porphyriacus* innocuous, yet he nevertheless included it within an ophidian genus replete with venomous species. Claiming that his original sample was damaged, by 1802 he received an intact specimen equipped with frontal fangs set apart from the line of subsequent teeth. Concurring with Buffon and Edward Gray that this dentition bespoke a venomous character, Shaw furthered his anatomical proof by noting that 'the animal is even said to be highly dreaded by the natives of Australasia'.[52] That same year he added the 'Antarctic boa' (*Acanthophis antarcticus*) to the catalogue of antipodean serpents, suggesting that it too was highly venomous but noting nothing of its fangs.[53]

In Sydney Town, Shaw's 'Antarctic boa' was initially named after the poisonous serpent of Psalm 58 – the wicked 'deaf adder that stoppeth her ear'. Soon tellingly corrupted to 'death adder', by 1804 this snake was 'supposed to be more fatal in its bite than any other' – albeit mainly because of its prominent fangs.[54] Concurrently, at the Muséum d'Histoire Naturelle, François Marie Daudin was also drawn to dentition in describing *Acanthophis antarcticus*, asking, 'Des crochets venimeux?'[55]

Anatomy and testimony, it seemed, were set against each other. In 1801, surgeon-explorer Matthew Flinders listed 'poisonous snakes' amongst the reptiles of Van Diemen's Land, but provided neither dental rationale nor witnessed evidence.[56] Yet while circumnavigating the island with Flinders in 1799, naval surgeon George Bass had attempted to capture a black snake 'with venomous fangs ... to try the effect of his bite upon a hawk we then had on board'.[57] Although frustrated by the death of the serpent – apparently poisoned by its own bite – this encounter comprised the first vivisection planned in the antipodes. It was on this same island colony, as Carol Freeman has shown, that visual and descriptive accounts of the thylacine saw it demonised as an antipodean 'wolf', justifying persecution for its presumptive depredations upon sheep.[58] Yet when it came to snakes, what was required by colonists was *active* proof that they were dangerous.

Snakes and ladders: the colonial animal matrix

While European naturalists and theologians sought to order new species from Australia into their proper place in nature, white colonists faced a more quotidian problem: determining where these creatures *belonged*. They responded by shuffling animals into three dynamic categories: useful, useless or noxious. Sometimes – especially when hungry – they sought advice from Aboriginal informants. Primarily, however, Europeans characterised autochthonous creatures in relation to other animals, especially the familiar beasts that co-colonised the continent alongside them.

Indeed, in the late eighteenth century, most Britons shared intimate, instrumental or occasionally sentimental relations with a menagerie of domesticated creatures.[59] It is no surprise that such beasts accompanied them wherever they ventured across the globe. Horses, oxen, cattle, goats, pigs, sheep, dogs, cats, rats, mice, bees, fowls, songbirds, foxes and rabbits proceeded ashore as autonomous beings. Other travellers, from barnacles to lice, detached themselves from settlers, their animals and their vessels at every site of occupation.[60]

Each colony thus evolved a unique yet dynamic series of equivalences and hierarchies between indigenous and immigrant animals. This matrix operated like the moralistic Hindu game, *vaikunthapaali*, later anglicised as 'snakes and ladders'. Horizontally layered tiers indicated equivalence, while vertical rows denoted hierarchies. Certain types might ascend the ladder of human estimation, whilst others slithered downward. Repositioning one creature often reshuffled the value ascribed to others. New entrants appeared with unanticipated consequences; others vanished forever through neglect or extermination.

Nominally biological descriptors such as 'native', 'wild' or 'vermin' rarely remained static within these Imperial ecologies.[61] Structuring animal relations also carried religious connotations, rationalising European notions of property as a divine mission of stewardship, as modelled in Figure 5. Rooted in specific locales, each colonial animal matrix codified commercial, sentimental and moral economies that were bound intimately – through tradition, trade and discourse – to multiple sites connected by intercolonial exchange. Each historically specific assemblage was shaped not just by human agency, but by geography, climate, technology, plants, diseases and the animals themselves.[62]

Australia was no exception. As James Boyce has convincingly argued, kangaroo-hunting dogs became critical to the survival of the first colonists in Van Diemen's Land.[63] By 1810 their utility as hunters, commodities and companions led to a vast increase in the social value

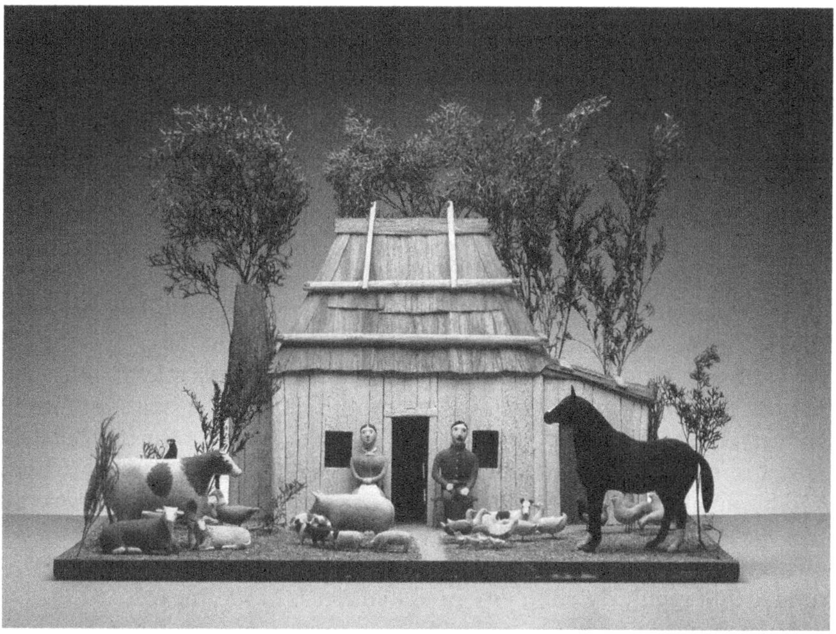

5 Charlotte Rushby, House model, early Australian settler's slab hut, *c.*1852.

of canines amongst settlers and Aborigines alike. In 1793 the registrar of the Vice-Admiralty Court in Sydney Town, Richard Atkins, recorded an epitaph for his favourite dog, whose 'heart, like thine, propell'd the crimson stream':

> Nature to him more liberal, 'tis true –
> He trod the earth on four thou only two
> From ancient blood of canine race he came
> Faithful he was, and Trusty was his name.[64]

Dogs were but one species amidst a menagerie of imported beasts. In 1788 British New South Wales comprised 990 humans, 200 fowls, 35 ducks, 29 geese, 18 turkeys, 5 rabbits, 49 pigs, 29 sheep, 6 horses, 4 cows, a bull and a calf. By 1800 there were more ungulates than colonists. Nevertheless, the duress of the voyage itself is often overlooked. Amongst a shipload of animals embarked for Sydney in 1793, all 24 cows, half of the 120 sheep, and the majority of 130 goats died on the journey.[65] The economic consequences were predictable. As Joan Goodrick has remarked, 'an animal was worth at least a human life, as those who indulged in sheep-stealing knew too well'.[66] Consequently, settlers remained closely attuned to accidents that might befall their beasts, from sheep scab to snakebite.

Breeds apart: wild dogs and Tasmanian tigers

Yet concern over the malleable morphology and domesticity of familiar animals proved disconcerting at the borderlines of 'wildness'. It was a common problem of empire; as geographer Kay Anderson observes, the 'metaphorical and technical faces of domestication ... hold up a mirror to tensions with the process of "human" self-definition in European-derived societies'.[67]

Such insecurities applied especially to the porous boundary between the indigenous dingo and the invading domestic dog, serving as an enduring synecdoche for Imperial concerns over racial miscegenation and atavism. 'Wild' dogs certainly caused the colonists more concern than poisonous serpents, chiefly on account of the danger they posed to other domesticates. Similarly, when a herd of cattle – which had escaped the Port Jackson settlement in 1788 – were rediscovered in 1795, they were considered too 'wild' to rejoin the colony's stocks. Of all imported quadrupeds, only horse breeding was carefully superintended and regularly supplemented by British bloodlines.[68]

If antipodean settlers struggled to control imported beasts, their shared status as invaders structured colonial relationships with Indigenous peoples and animals alike. As in colonial America, New

Zealand and South Africa, sheep, cattle and swine served as 'empire's proxy', literally and legally occupying a presumptive *terra nullius*.[69] This economic – and thus political – imperative proved a potent tool for Aboriginal dispossession, an othering process which sustained the colonisers' identification with their familiar quadrupeds. While Indigenous Australians were punished – often lethally – for killing livestock, the primary threat to colonising animals was four-legged. On the mainland dingoes became 'a fearful scourge to the settlers on the large sheep-runs'; in Van Diemen's Land the thylacine was systematically eradicated as 'vermin' largely due to its supposed slaughter of settler sheep.[70] By 1820, such conjunctions had likewise positioned Australian snakes at the bottom of the colonial animal matrix.

Surmising the snakebite syndrome, 1788–1820

In the decades after 1788, animals killed few white settlers: the first deaths attributed to fauna were three soldiers who drowned when a whale overturned their boat in Sydney Harbour in 1790. Even as occupation expanded to Van Diemen's Land, snakebite remained an apparently rare occurrence. In 1827, visiting naval surgeon Peter Cunningham remarked that 'comparatively few deaths [have] taken place from this cause since the foundation of the colony'.[71] Twenty years later, settler Alexander Harris reaffirmed that 'It is a circumstance which elicits a universal expression of surprise among the colonists that, snakes being so common as they are, so few persons should be bitten.'[72]

Indeed, Australian snakes were at first presumed innocent. In 1793, marine Lieutenant Watkin Tench related three competing strands of testimony: settler experience, Aboriginal behaviour and observation of the effects in a familiar animal:

> Of snakes there are two or three sorts: but whether the bite of any of them be mortal, or even venomous, is somewhat doubtful. I know of but one well attested instance of a bite being received from a snake. A soldier was bitten so as to draw blood, and the wound healed as a simple incision does without showing any symptom of malignity. A dog was *reported* to be bitten by a snake, and the animal swelled and died in great agony. But I will by no means affirm that the cause of his death was fairly ascertained. It is, however, certain that the natives show on all occasions the utmost horror of the snake.[73]

Opportunities for such observations soon multiplied. Recounting the first settler death involving an affray with a local snake in January

1792, Governor David Collins was adamant: the cause was not 'any effect of the bite of the snake, but from a general debility'. As serpents grew more prominent, however, Collins became less forgiving. When a convict was bitten by a black snake in Sydney Town in January 1795, the colony's assistant surgeon, James Thompson, 'saved the man's life without having recourse to amputation'. That March, a woman bitten at Prospect Hill was likewise rescued by the ministrations of convict surgeon John Irving.[74] The first snakebite death Collins reported was a man at the Hawkesbury River in November 1795, while a woman 'died of the bite of a snake' in the same locality in 1798. Amidst the 2326 souls interred at the Old Sydney Burial Ground was Samuel Allgate, 'Killed by a snake' on 3 March 1802.[75]

Indeed, by that date Australian serpents were being depicted as 'highly poisonous' both within the colony and in European natural history texts. Justifications came as much from animal victims as humans. On 9 October 1793, Atkins noted that while it had 'been imagined [that] the Snakes of this country are not venemous, we are now convinced to the Contrary'. His evidence: when a black snake bit two chickens belonging to the colony's master carpenter, one 'died in 1½ minutes, another in 2 minutes'.[76] In December 1803, the continent's inaugural newspaper ran its first snakebite report: setting upon a 'very large black snake', a terrier 'only outlived his antagonist a few minutes'.[77] The following year, a valuable hound was bitten by a 'viper'; 'seized suddenly with a hydrophobia', the dog died within five minutes.[78] This case seamlessly corroborated the *Sydney Gazette*'s first reported human fatality on 15 October 1804, when 11-year-old John Howorth 'received a bite from a black snake', fell into a stupor and died within twelve hours (Figure 6).[79]

Howorth's death from a 'subtle surpents Bite' spurred an upsurge in snakebite reports over 1804–05. Two months later a sheep was found dead near Parramatta, with foam in its nostrils and a puncture on its lip. That month the *Sydney Gazette* condemned the 'black snake principally dreaded by the stock-keeper as the chief, if not the only member of the reptile order dangerous to his charge'.[80] Larger animals were not immune; in 1806 a bullock – worth perhaps £25 – suffered a painful demise following a bite. By 1809 unexplained deaths in horses and cows were being credibly attributed to snakebite.

As early as 1805 a syndrome of symptoms was imputed to bites by Australian snakes, being seamlessly extrapolated across animal species and into humans. In 1805, for instance, a Sydney shepherd was considered lucky to have survived a bite from a 'black snake' that had fatally bitten one of his lambs. Less fortunate was James Swift in 1807; surviving but 25 minutes, his case was the first reported deadly

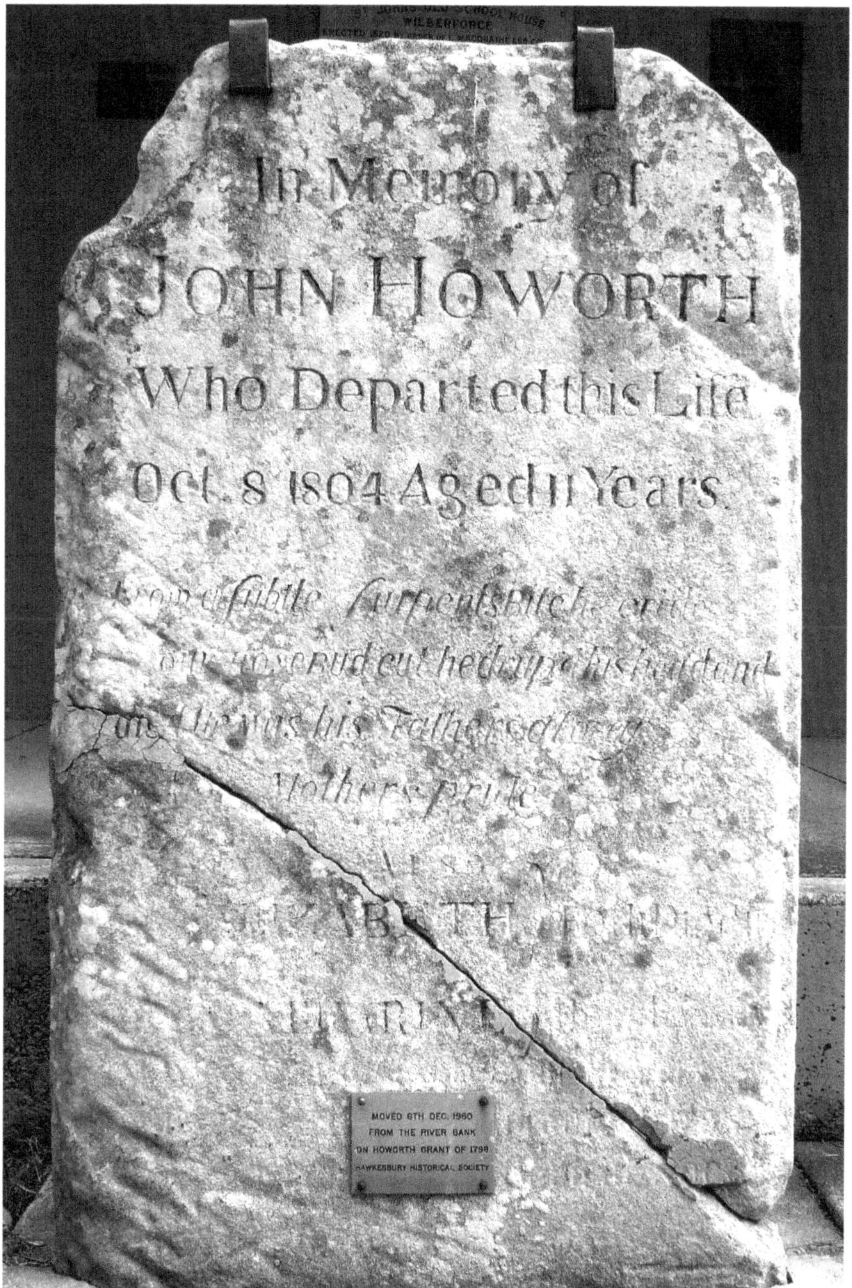
In Memory of
JOHN HOWORTH
Who Departed this Life
Oct. 8 1804 Aged 11 Years
MOVED 6TH DEC. 1960
FROM THE RIVER BANK
ON HOWORTH GRANT OF 1798
HAWKESBURY HISTORICAL SOCIETY

6 Headstone of John Howorth, 1804, St John's Churchyard, Wilberforce, New South Wales.

snakebite in Van Diemen's Land.[81] In 1808, 13-year-old William Nash became possibly the first locally born colonist to die from snakebite. Little wonder that in 1810, surgeon Joseph Arnold wrote that Sydney's inland regions abounded 'in many kinds of dangerous serpents, the bites of which are instant death'.[82]

Reinforcing the human–animal link, in 1814 the *Sydney Gazette* blamed a 'black snake' for the demise of John Kenny, because a 'day or two previously the unfortunate subject of this melancholy report had had two favorite [*sic*] dogs killed in the same manner, as from every symptom attending the death of the animals was undoubted'.[83] When John Wood of the Royal Veteran Company died after a bite at Bathurst two years later, the case was considered closed when a sheep bitten nearby displayed identical signs: instant death and rapid putrescence.[84]

In Van Diemen's Land, *The Hobart Town Gazette and Southern Reporter* ran five accounts of snakebite over its first half-decade of publication from 1816. That December a hen was killed by a four-foot 'black snake', followed in 1819 by 14-month-old Elizabeth Lowe.[85] The mainland, nevertheless, remained the main arena. In 1815 John Moore, aged 15, died following a bite by 'a yellow snake'. He first 'complained of thirst; and after drinking some milk, was seized with a vomiting'. Subsequently losing his vision, Moore's 'speech was also much affected, and he articulated his words with difficulty ... his tongue [was] yellow and much swelled, and his teeth black'.[86] Despite a revival, the youth passed away in Sydney Hospital 24 hours after the bite.

Based upon such sketchy and incomplete records, over 1795–1819 at least 18 human fatalities could be attributed to snakebite in New South Wales, plus two in Van Diemen's Land – approximately one death per annum. A third of the victims were 15 years or younger. Concurrently, since 1788 snakebite had accounted for at least six dogs, four sheep, two cattle, a horse and a handful of fowls, although many veterinary cases likely remained unreported.

Identifying the responsible ophidian rarely required a naturalist: to the colonists all that mattered was size and colour. In his 1813 manuscript of natural history, for instance, Thomas Skottowe drew five local serpents, noting that 'These Noxious Reptiles are all venomous. The Black Snake is however the Worst, its bite being almost instantaneously Mortal.'[87] Certainly black snakes – with or without crimson bellies – were the most commonly reported variety, but settlers also observed yellow, brown, blue, green, grey or diamond serpents. Moreover, all were believed to possess fangs. '[I]n this colony we have never yet heard that any have been seen without those deadly weapons of defence', summarised the *Sydney Gazette* in 1817, 'and therefore must infer that all are poisonous in a greater or inferior degree'.[88]

Brute creation and plebeian expertise

By the 1820s, serpents were no longer the innocent creatures of White and Tench. Not only did an 'offending reptile' attack Elizabeth Hartley; when chased by an axe-wielding servant, 'the animal turned on him, as if conscious of the necessity of executing its fatal powers in self-defence'.[89] In 1824 Australian ophidians were portrayed as serving 'an allwise purpose which is to quell human pride, and repress the boasts of security'.[90] Indeed domestic spaces – as much as domestic species – were threatened by home invasions from snakes seeking shelter, fowls and rodents. Silent serpents may have been but, in the words of Jennifer Martin, they were also undeniably 'historical subjects with their own agency-in-the-world'.[91]

Moreover, by 1820 both popular discourse and medical opinion concurred that a characteristic set of signs and symptoms followed snakebite in human and non-human victims alike. This knowledge remained particularly parochial. Although adopting the familiar nomenclature of snakes, vipers and adders, settlers rarely invoked British, American or Indian species. Australian serpents were known primarily on their own terms, especially black snakes which were generally regarded as lethal.[92]

Naturalists, indeed, proved peripheral to Australian understanding of indigenous serpents. In 1841 the *Sydney Gazette* warned immigrants that New South Wales teemed with 'snakes of different kinds and adders, all venomous, their bite is fatal, unless remedies are used without delay'.[93] But how was such local expertise generated? Eschewing anatomy for testimony, settlers circulated knowledge about snakebite and its treatment well beyond the formal networks of natural history which, into the 1850s, were confined to rarefied society.[94] Published in 1837, the first catalogue of the new Australian Museum in Sydney merely noted 'Ten specimens' of snakes, offering neither names nor an assessment of their noxiousness.[95] Visiting zoologists such as Charles Darwin added even less, even as their collections swelled with Australian specimens.

Indeed, the settlers' chief informants were not naturalists, but animal familiars. An intimate part of almost every household, imported beasts populated streets, yards and fields. Scampering unseen into granaries, storehouses and pantries, they shared journeys by road or across trackless territory. Against the rarity of human fatalities, by 1820 the proliferation of animal cases engendered comparisons across species, from cat to cow, dog to ram. Thereby the colonists registered a snakebite syndrome including vomiting, lassitude, staggering, creeping paralysis, collapse, agonised expiry and putrescent swelling. These homologies held into the human species.

Horror redoubled: entrenching snakes in the colonial animal matrix

From the 1790s into the 1830s, dogs remained the bellwether of colonial concern over snakebite. In his popular 1827 account, Cunningham detailed this danger via a narrative of two canine companions, 'a fine pointer newly from England, and the other a colonial-bred kangaroo dog'.[96] With both soon acquiring the habit of confronting snakes, their fates during an excursion into the bush resembled a fable. The pointer was bitten first; its fate was sealed. A second bite then accounted for the kangaroo dog, which became paralysed in the hind legs, then the forequarters, before suffering a seizure and expiring within half an hour. Both canine corpses bloated markedly after death. 'Dogs are the greatest sufferers', affirmed William Leigh, visiting Kangaroo Island in 1839. Amazed that more settlers were not bitten by the abundant snakes, he remarked the 'tremendous mortality' among dogs, 'a large hound living after the bite but seven or eight minutes, and swelling up like a tun [barrel]'.[97]

Direct extrapolations across species were frequent and overt. In 1836, William Govett detailed the galloping demise of one of his favoured hunting dogs. Bitten by a 'large gray snake' – which Govett's Aboriginal companions asserted was deadly – 'Duke' gave an unearthly shriek and collapsed. Soon, 'the whole of the inside of his mouth, was choked with a thick and clammy white foam … before I could examine him, the animal reeled a few paces between us, like a drunken man, and fell dead!' Noting that sheep and cattle suffered similar fates, Govett recoiled: 'how must this horror be redoubled to witness the effects of the venom upon a human being!'[98]

Thus was the evidence ever before the settlers' eyes. Explorer Hamilton Hume recounted a snakebite in the widely read narrative of his 1824 expedition. Bitten on the nose by a 'yellow snake', one of his horses died within twenty minutes. Found 'with its body blown up, and bleeding from the nostrils', it appeared that a similar cause despatched one of Ludwig Leichhardt's expedition ponies in 1845.[99] Although more explorers in nineteenth-century Australia were killed by their camels, mules and horses than by serpents, it was clear which creature alarmed man and beast alike.

Founded upon such equivalences, an animal matrix emerged in the Australian colonies. While the harshness of early settler life may have predicated against sentimental attachment to livestock, the enormous value accorded to domesticates heightened awareness of their ailments. Furthermore, as conjoint invaders, British beasts and colonisers were united against indigenous foes, whether Aboriginal or animal. In extrapolating the symptoms of snakebite across familiar species, the colonists furthermore situated themselves on the same animal spectrum as sheep, horses, cattle and canines. Soon enough, settlers determined that direct observation of deliberate snakebite in familiar animals – especially dogs – offered an effective indicator.

After 1840 this practice – termed 'vivisection' in contemporary Europe – emerged as a new thread of active inquiry in the colonial antipodes. As with cases of accidental snakebite, staged experiments soon became so commonplace as to escape comment. One corollary was a moral indifference to the suffering of animals unwillingly enlisted for such spectacles. Another was the effect of popular demand for these demonstrations on colonial medical epistemology. Underlying all of these performances was the ambiguous relationship between snakes and their enigmatic animal fluid, venom.

Notes

1 William Romaine Govett, *Sketches of New South Wales* (Melbourne: Gaston Renard, 1977), p. 40.

2 Richard Bowler, 'Broadmarsh, Tasmania', in Eric Rolls (ed.), *Visions of Australia: Impressions of the Landscape 1642–1910* (South Melbourne: Thomas C. Lothian, 2002), p. 126.

3 See George Basalla, 'The spread of Western science', *Science*, 156:3775 (1967), pp. 611–22; Roy MacLeod, 'On visiting the "moving metropolis": reflections on the architecture of imperial science', *Historical Records of Australian Science*, 5:3 (1980), pp. 1–16; Jan Todd, 'Science at the periphery: an interpretation of Australian scientific and technological dependency and development prior to 1914', *Annals of Science*, 50:1 (1993), pp. 33–58.

4 M.E. Hoare, 'Doctor John Henderson and the Van Diemen's Land Scientific Society', *Records of the Australian Academy of Science*, 1:3 (1966), pp. 7–24; Jan Kociumbas, 'Science as cultural ideology: museums and mechanics' institutes in early New South Wales and Van Diemen's Land', *Labour History*, 64 (1993), pp. 17–33.

5 'History of water snakes, sea snakes, and sea serpents', *The Australian Magazine*, I:1 (1821), pp. 15–18.

6 Erica Fudge, *Perceiving Animals: Humans and Beasts in Early Modern English Culture* (Urbana: University of Illinois Press, 2002), pp. 93–7.

7 King James version.

8 Esther Cohen, 'Animals in medieval perceptions: the image of the ubiquitous other', in Aubrey Manning and James Serpell (eds), *Animals and Human Society: Changing Perspectives* (London: Routledge, 1994), pp. 60–1.

9 See Brunsdon Yapp and Wilma George, 'Other animals', in Wilma George and Brunsdon Yapp (eds), *The Naming of Beasts: Natural History in the Medieval Bestiary* (London: Duckworth, 1991), pp. 190–202.

10 Edward Topsell, *The Historie of Serpents* (London: William Jaggard, 1608), p. 37.

11 A.R., *True and Wonderfull a Discourse Relating to a Strange and Monstrous Serpent (or Dragon) Lately Discouered* (London: Iohn Trundle, 1614), title page.

12 Topsell, *The Historie of Serpents*, p. 42.

13 *Ibid.*, p. 40.

14 Kathleen Walker-Meikle, 'Toxicology and treatment: medical authorities and snake-bite in the middle ages', *Korot*, 22 (2013–14), p. 93.

15 Daniel Sennert, Nicholas Culpeper, and Abdiah Cole, *The Sixth Book of Practical Physick of Occult or Hidden Diseases* (London: Peter Cole, 1662), pp. 67–9.

16 Jutta Schickore, 'Trying again and again: multiple repetitions in early modern reports of experiments on snake bites', *Early Science and Medicine*, 15:6 (2010), pp. 578–9.

17 Moyse Charas, *New Experiments Upon Vipers Containing Also an Exact Description of All the Parts of a Viper, the Seat of Its Poyson, and the Several Effects Thereof* (London: J. Martyn, 1670), preface, p. 93.

18 *Ibid.*, p. 138; Henry Stubbe, *An Epistolary Discourse Concerning Phlebotomy in Opposition to G. Thomson Pseudo-Chymist, a Pretended Disciple of the Lord Verulam* (London, 1671), pp. 10–11. Italics in original.

19 Francesco Redi, *A Letter of Francesco Redi Concerning Some Objections Made Upon His Observations about Vipers Written to Monsieur Bourdelot, Abbott, and Lord of Conde and St. Leger and Monsieur Alexander Morus* (London: John Martyn, 1673), pp. 6–7.

20 Jay Tribby, 'Cooking (with) Clio and Cleo: eloquence and experiment in seventeenth-century Florence', *Journal of the History of Ideas*, 52:3 (1991), p. 423.

21 Schickore, 'Trying again and again', p. 580.

22 Martha Baldwin, 'The snakestone experiments: an early modern medical debate', *Isis*, 86:3 (1995), pp. 414–18.

23 See for instance Ramya Raman, Anantanarayanan Raman and P. Ram Manohar, 'The arsenic and mercury-containing tanjore pills used in treating snake bites in the 18th century Madras presidency', *Current Science*, 106:12 (2014), pp. 1759–63.

24 Richard Mead, *A Mechanical Account of Poisons, in Several Essays*, 5th (corrected) edn (London: J. Brindley, 1756), pp. xxix, xxxi.

25 Walter Sneader, *Drug Discovery: A History* (Chichester: John Wiley & Sons, 2005), pp. 41–6.

26 Daniel Turner, *De Morbis Cutaneis. A Treatise of Diseases Incident to the Skin*, 5th (corrected) edn (London: R. Wilkin, J. and J. Bonwicke, S. Birt, T. Ward and E. Wicksteed, 1736), p. 398. Italics in original.

27 R. Brookes, *The General Practice of Physic*, 5th edn, vol. 2 (London: J. Newbery, 1765), p. 154. Italics in original.

28 Stanford Wolsterstan, *An Enquiry Into the Causes of Diseases in General and the Disturbances of the Humors in Man's Body Wherein the Nature of the Blood, of the Air and of a Pestiliential Constitution Are Briefly Considered* (London: Thomas Basset, 1692), pp. 51–2.

29 Peter Shaw, *A New Practice of Physic*, 7th (corrected) edn, vol. I (London: T. and T. Longman, 1753), p. 193.

30 Henry Baker, *The Microscope Made Easy*, 5th edn (London: J. Dodsley, 1769), p. 214.

31 Georges Louis Leclerc Buffon, *Natural History: General and Particular*, vol. 2 (Edinburgh: William Creech, 1780), p. 348.

32 Christiane Nockels Fabbri, 'Treating medieval plague: the wonderful virtues of theriac', *Early Science and Medicine*, 12:3 (2007), pp. 252–4.

33 James Handley, *Mechanical Essays On the Animal Oeconomy* (London: A. Bettesworth and C. Rivington, 1721), p. 301. Italics in original.

34 Pratik Chakrabarti, *Materials and Medicine: Trade, Conquest and Therapeutics in the Eighteenth Century* (Manchester: Manchester University Press, 2010), p. 198.

35 See Projit Bihari Mukharji, 'Pharmacology, "indigenous knowledge", nationalism: a few words from the epitaph of subaltern science', in Mark Harrison and Biswamoy Pati (eds), *The Social History of Health and Medicine in Colonial India* (London: Routledge, 2009), pp. 201–2, and David Arnold, 'The politics of poison: healing, empowerment and subversion in nineteenth-century India', in David Hardiman and Projit Bihari Mukharji (eds), *Medical Marginality in South Asia: Situating Subaltern Therapeutics* (Abingdon: Routledge, 2012), pp. 171–92.

36 Guy Attewell, 'Interweaving substance trajectories: tiryaq, circulation and therapeutic transformation in the nineteenth century', in Anne Digby, Waltraud Ernst and Projit B. Mukharji (eds), *Crossing Colonial Historiographies: Histories of*

Colonial and Indigenous Medicines in Transnational Perspective (Newcastle upon Tyne: Cambridge Scholars Publishing, 2010), p. 13.

37 William King, *An Essay On the Origin of Evil*, 2nd edn, vol. I (London: W. Thurlbourn, 1732), p. 206.

38 Charles Owen, *An Essay Towards a Natural History of Serpents* (London: Charles Owen, 1742), p. 43.

39 *Beauties of Natural History; Or, Elements of Zoography* (London: Richardson and Urquhart, 1777), p. 94.

40 Captain Hall, 'An account of some experiments on the effects of the poison of the rattle-snake', *Philosophical Transactions: Giving Some Account of the Present Undertakings, Studies and Labours of the Ingenious in Many Considerable Parts of the World*, vol. 34 (1728), p. 352.

41 Mead, *A Mechanical Account of Poisons*, p. 41.

42 Thomas R. Dunlap, *Nature and the English Diaspora: Environment and History in the United States, Canada, Australia, and New Zealand* (Cambridge: Cambridge University Press, 1999), pp. 44–5.

43 Mary Elizabeth Leighton and Lisa Surridge, 'The empire bites back: the racialised crocodile of the nineteenth century', in Deborah Denenholz Morse and Martin A. Danahay (eds), *Victorian Animal Dreams: Representations of Animals in Victorian Literature and Culture* (Aldershot: Ashgate, 2007), pp. 253, 255.

44 Mark V. Barrow Jr, 'The alligator's allure: changing perceptions of a charismatic carnivore', in Dorothee Brantz, ed., *Beastly Natures: Animals, Humans, and the Study of History* (Charlottesville: University of Virginia Press, 2010), p. 133.

45 Harriet Ritvo, 'Beasts in the jungle (or wherever)', *Daedalus*, 137:2 (2008), p. 25.

46 Samuel Ward, *A Modern System of Natural History*, vol. 11 (London: F. Newbery, 1775–76), p. 89. Italics in original.

47 Georges Louis Leclerc Buffon, *Natural History of Birds, Fish, Insects and Reptiles* (London: J.S. Barr, 1793), pp. 88–9.

48 Oliver Goldsmith, *An History of the Earth, and Animated Nature*, 2nd edn, vol. 7 (London: J. Nourse, 1779), p. 197.

49 *Ibid.*, pp. 159–60.

50 John White, *Journal of a Voyage To New South Wales With Sixty-Five Plates of Non Descript Animals, Birds, Lizards, Serpents, Curious Cones of Trees and Other Natural Productions* (London: I. Debrett, 1790), pp. 258–9.

51 Christoph Christian Sturm, *Reflections for Every Day in the Year, on the Works of God, and of His Providence Throughout All Nature*, 7th edn, vol. 2 (Edinburgh: N.R. Cheyne, 1800), p. 90.

52 George Shaw, *General Zoology; Or Systematic Natural History*, vol. 2, part II (London: G. Kearsley, 1802), pp. 423–4, 505–6.

53 George Shaw and E.R. Nodder, *Naturalist's Miscellany*, vol. 13 (London: Nodder & Co., 1802), Plate 535.

54 'Sydney', *Sydney Gazette and New South Wales Advertiser* (30 December 1804), p. 2.

55 F.M. Daudin, *Histoire Naturelle, Générale et Particulière des Reptiles* (Paris: F. Dufart, 1803 [Année XI]), p. 287.

56 Matthew Flinders, *Observations On the Coasts of Van Diemen's Land, On Bass's Strait and Its Islands, and On Part of the Coasts of New South Wales* (London: John Nichols, 1801), p. 21.

57 Dan Sprod (ed.), *Van Diemen's Land Revealed: Flinders and Bass and Their Circumnavigation of the Island in the Colonial Sloop Norfolk 1798–1799* (Hobart: Blubber Head Press, 2009), p. 82.

58 Carol Freeman, *Paper Tiger: A Visual History of the Thylacine* (Leiden: Brill, 2010), pp. 117–41.

59 See for instance Robert Malcolmson and Stephanos Mastoris, *The English Pig: A History* (London: Hambledon and London, 1998), p. 29.

60 Alfred W. Crosby, *Ecological Imperialism: The Biological Expansion of Europe, 900–1900* (Cambridge: Cambridge University Press, 1986), pp. 172–87.

61 Ritvo, 'Beasts in the jungle', pp. 22–30.

62 See Tim Ingold, 'From trust to domination: an alternative history of human–animal relations', in Aubrey Manning and James Serpell (eds), *Animals and Human Society: Changing Perspectives* (London: Routledge, 1994), pp. 1–22; William S. Lynn, 'Animals, ethics, and geography', in Jennifer Wolch and Jody Emel (eds), *Animal Geographies: Place, Politics, and Identity in the Nature–Culture Borderlands* (London: Verso, 1998), pp. 288–90.

63 James Boyce, 'A dog's breakfast … lunch and dinner: canine dependency in early Van Diemen's Land', *Tasmanian Historical Research Association Papers and Proceedings*, 51:4 (2004), pp. 194–213.

64 National Library of Australia, Canberra, MS 4039, Richard Atkins, 'Journal of Richard Atkins', 1791–1810, p. 26.

65 David Collins, *An Account of the English Colony in New South Wales: With Remarks On the Dispositions, Customs, Manners, &c. of the Native Inhabitants of That Country*, vol. I (London: T. Cadell Jun. and W. Davies, 1798), p. 270.

66 Joan Goodrick, *Life in Old Van Diemens Land* (London: Robert Hale, 1978), p. 115.

67 Kay Anderson, 'A walk on the wild side: a critical geography of domestication', *Progress in Human Geography*, 21:4 (1997), p. 473.

68 Ian Parsonson, *The Australian Ark: A History of Domesticated Animals in Australia* (Collingwood: CSIRO Publishing, 2000), pp. 120–2.

69 Leigh Dale, 'Empire's proxy: sheep and the colonial environment', in Helen Tiffin (ed.), *Five Emus to the King of Siam: Environment and Empire* (Amsterdam: Rodopi, 2007), pp. 9–11; Virginia DeJohn Anderson, *Creatures of Empire: How Domestic Animals Transformed Early America* (Oxford: Oxford University Press, 2004), pp. 160–71, 211–16.

70 An Old Bushman, *Bush Wanderings of a Naturalist; or, Notes on the Field Sports and Fauna of Australia Felix* (London: Routledge, Warne, & Routledge, 1861), pp. 36–7; Freeman, *Paper Tiger*, pp. 65–8, 107–8.

71 Peter Cunningham, *Two Years in New South Wales*, 2nd edn, vol. I (Sydney: Angus and Robertson in association with the Royal Australian Historical Society, 1966), p. 165.

72 An Emigrant Mechanic, *Settlers and Convicts: Or Recollections of Sixteen Years' Labour in the Australian Backwoods* (Carlton: Melbourne University Press, 1969), p. 146.

73 Watkin Tench, *1788: Comprising a Narrative of the Expedition to Botany Bay and a Complete Account of the Settlement at Port Jackson* (Melbourne: Text Publishing, 1996), pp. 242–3. Italics in original.

74 Collins, *An Account of the English Colony in New South Wales, Vol. I*, pp. 197–8, 404, 415.

75 Lisa Murray, 'Old Sydney Burial Ground', *Phanfare: Newsletter of the Professional Historians' Association (NSW)*, p. 228 (January–February 2008), p. 7.

76 Journal of Richard Atkins, p. 9 October 1793.

77 'Sydney', *Sydney Gazette and New South Wales Advertiser* (11 December 1803), p. 4.

78 'Sydney', *Sydney Gazette and New South Wales Advertiser* (21 October 1804), p. 3.

79 *Ibid.*

80 *Ibid.*, p. 2.

81 'Sydney', *Sydney Gazette and New South Wales Advertiser* (22 February 1807), p. 2.

82 Martin, *A New Land*, p. 87.

83 'Sydney', *Sydney Gazette and New South Wales Advertiser* (12 February 1814), p. 2.

84 'Sydney', *Sydney Gazette and New South Wales Advertiser* (24 February 1816), p. 2.

85 'Hobart Town', *Hobart Town Gazette and Southern Reporter* (20 February 1819), p. 2.

86 'Sydney', *Sydney Gazette and New South Wales Advertiser* (23 December 1815), p. 2.

87 State Library of New South Wales, Sydney, PXA 555, Thomas Skottowe, 'Select

Specimens From Nature of the Birds Animals &c &c of New South Wales', 1813, p. 53.

88 'Sydney', *Sydney Gazette and New South Wales Advertiser* (3 May 1817), p. 3.

89 'Sydney', *Sydney Gazette and New South Wales Advertiser* (3 April 1819), pp. 2–3.

90 'Police office news', *Sydney Gazette and New South Wales Advertiser* (18 November 1824), p. 3.

91 Jennifer Adams Martin, 'When sharks (don't) attack: wild animal agency in historical narratives', *Environmental History*, 16:3 (2011), p. 455.

92 R.-P. Lesson, *Voyage Autour du Monde Exécuté par Ordre du Roi, sur la Corvette de sa Majesté, La Coquille* (Paris: Arthus Bertrand, 1832), p. 30.

93 'An Australian', 'Sketch of Australia', *Sydney Gazette and New South Wales Advertiser* (16 October 1841), p. 5.

94 See Nick Drayson, 'Early developments in the literature of Australian natural history: together with a select bibliography of Australian natural history writing, printed in English, from 1697 to the present' (PhD thesis, Australian Defence Force Academy, University of New South Wales, 1997), pp. 25–30.

95 Australian Museum, *A Catalogue of the Specimens of Natural History and Miscellaneous Curiosities Deposited in the Australian Museum* (Sydney: James Tegg, 1837), p. 59.

96 Cunningham, *Two Years in New South Wales*, p. 164.

97 W.H. Leigh, *Reconnoitering Voyages and Travels, with Adventures in the New Colonies of South Australia* (Milson's Point: Currawong Press, 1982), p. 97.

98 Govett, *Sketches of New South Wales*, p. 42.

99 Ludwig Leichhardt, *Journal of an Overland Expedition in Australia, from Moreton Bay to Port Essington, a Distance of Upwards of 3000 Miles, during the Years 1844–1845* (North Adelaide: Corkwood Press, 2000), p. 191.

CHAPTER TWO

Vivisection in the pub: public spectacles and plebeian expertise, 1840–80

As knowledge of Australian serpents began to stabilise by 1820, settler correspondence increasingly referred to 'the usual remedies' for snakebite. What was 'usual', however, proved remarkably diverse. Until the 1840s, almost all treatments arose from received knowledge: European folklore, Aboriginal informants or medical dictums. Thereafter, a new and more potent source emerged: animals. Public demonstrations of snakebite in living creatures became the central device through which Australian colonists determined the deadliest serpents and the most efficacious antidotes. In short, they embraced the practice and epistemology of vivisection.

This widespread adoption of animal experimentation had enduring moral and heuristic corollaries. First, because snakebite demonstrations were conducted upon domesticated species, their popularity both signified and strengthened the Europeans' identification with their animal familiars. The associated ethical questions, however, only rarely entered public discourse. Second, as this chapter argues, antipodean uptake of vivisection was not driven by doctors. Such was the public acceptance of snake showmen and antidote sellers that until the 1870s, clinicians and scientists were impelled to emulate – or collaborate with – plebeian experts.

In contrast to the prevailing teleology of natural history, this 'vivisection in the pub' represented a challenge to the uncertain legitimacy of colonial doctors and natural philosophers. Within settler societies negotiating a wider franchise and jury service, snakebite spectacles echoed the 1819 New York court case in which naturalists testified that whales were *not* fish. As Graham Burnett argues in *Trying Leviathan*, this episode presented 'a gloriously feisty public forum where competing parties deployed a wide range of skills, texts, and authorities in efforts to undermine (and sometimes undergird) the edifice of contemporary taxonomy'.[1] Amidst the competing parties – gentleman naturalists, lay experts, commercial stakeholders and credulous publics – such resources of proof remained highly mobile.

The Grand Elixir: the colonial quest for a snakebite antidote

Although public vivisection was not unique to the Australian colonies, in the Victorian era it was rare to find an insistence on animal experimentation so prominently foregrounded. Included in poet 'Banjo' Paterson's phenomenally popular *The Man from Snowy River and Other Verses* (1895) – which sold 7000 copies within a month – was 'Johnson's Antidote'. Seeking a cure for snakebite – 'the Grand Elixir, greatest blessing ever known' – the eponymous William Johnson consults an Aboriginal man. 'King Billy' directs Johnson to watch a contest between two indigenous creatures: a goanna and tiger snake. When the lizard emerges triumphant but then nibbles a nearby bush, Johnson presumes it a natural snakebite remedy. He rushes to the local museum where, advising against auto-experimentation, a 'scientific man' suggests instead:

> Get a pair of dogs and try it, let the snake give both a nip;
> Give your dog the snakebite mixture, let the other fellow rip.

While another hound and Johnson's faithful 'Stumpy' both receive the venom of a deadly snake, only the latter is given Johnson's Antidote. Sadly, only 'Stumpy' ends up 'as dead as mutton', prompting the scientist to hurriedly conduct further tests:

> Half a tumbler killed an emu, half a spoonful killed a goat,
> All the snakes on earth were harmless to that awful antidote.[2]

Paterson's poem neatly encapsulated the multiple modes of proletarian antidote science across nineteenth-century Australia. Dismissive of Aboriginal knowledge, yet convinced that the local environment would furnish a cure, the settlers turned to animals. Given the goanna's reputed imperviousness to snakebite, they trusted this lizard to guide them to lucrative 'secret' herbs. Above all, settlers relied upon – indeed, demanded – animal experiments to prove the potency of snake venom and the efficacy of antidotes. Whether conducted in public houses or public institutions, the sacrifice of domestic animals for these trials was frequent and blatant, yet morally unproblematic. 'Stumpy' was no fiction, and he was far from alone.

But dead dogs were never the settlers' only guide (Figures 7 and 8). European medicine, folklore and natural theology endured well into the 1860s. An early trope was divine beneficence or natural balance: the presumption that the Maker might provide an antidote in the

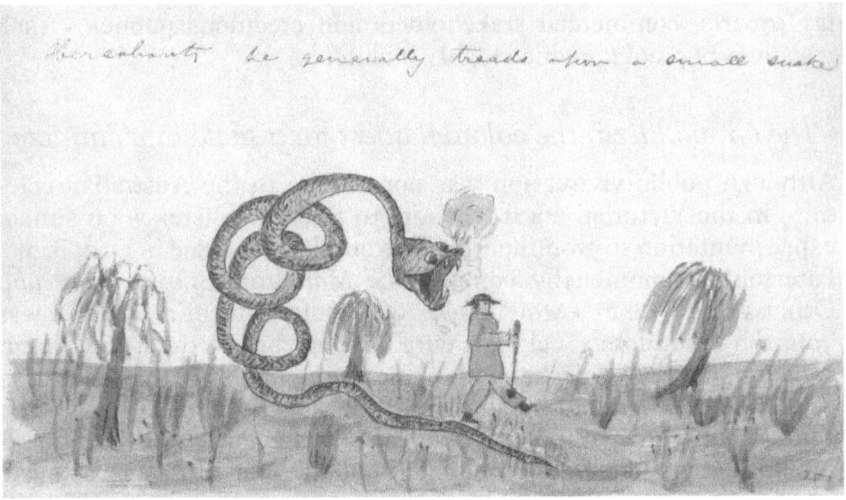

7 Edward Wilson, 'Hereabouts he generally treads upon a small snake', *c.*1842–78.

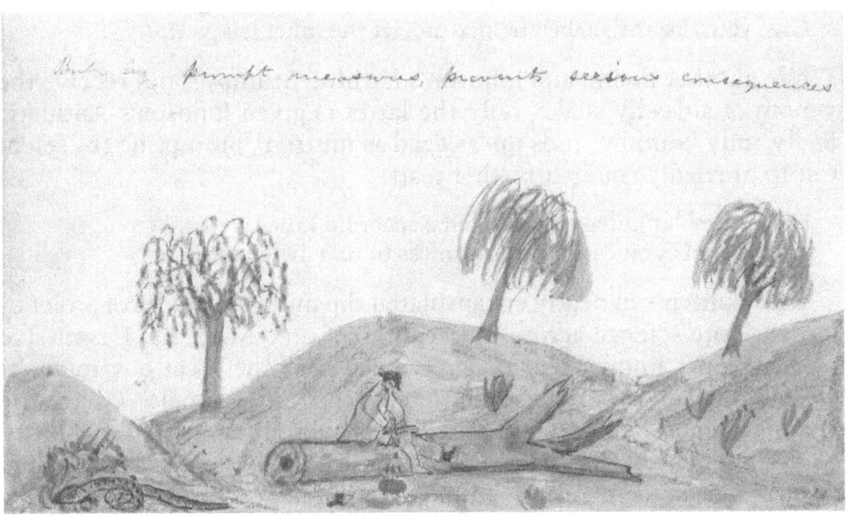

8 Edward Wilson, 'But by prompt measures, prevents serious consequences', *c.*1842–78.

local environment, or within the snake itself, underlay a host of 'cures'. Whether revealed by providence, Aboriginal informants or local animals, however, the active element usually remained a closely guarded secret.

Another potent European tradition was theriac. Originating in antiquity, this complex preparation gained repute as an alexipharmic – a universal antidote. Serving first to remedy the bites of wild or venomous beasts, theriac transmogrified into mithridatium, claimed to neutralise all poisons. In the Roman world, Galen verified his variant of 'theriaca' via vivisection.[3] Frequently comprising 50 to 80 herbal and animal ingredients – including opium and viper flesh – by 1700, its preparation constituted a ceremonial activity involving whole communities, often sustaining a substantial commercial economy. In Britain, however, its fortunes waned by the mid-eighteenth century. Commonly known as 'treacle', theriac was expunged from the London Pharmacopœia in 1746 and its Edinburgh equivalent by 1752.[4] It has been speculated that in the Australian colonies, 'the sulphur and treacle mixture, administered to so many pioneer children, was a debased Theriaca'.[5]

Perhaps the prime reason for theriac's decline was a British medical insistence on 'simples'. Theriac typified not just the complexity of Galenic dogma, but its allopathic rationale. After 1700, this reliance upon opposing actions was increasingly challenged by a Paracelsian insistence on similars: like curing like. The recognition and application of single, pure agents targeted to their appropriate malady remained central to the training of British physicians and apothecaries until the mid-nineteenth century.[6] Immediately they arrived on colonial shores, therefore, British-trained healers experimented with Australian flora, seeking botanical equivalents of familiar simples.[7]

Doctors were not the only dispensers. By the 1820s, snakebitten settlers in New South Wales would cut out the bitten part and apply a poultice of chewed herbs. Surgeon Peter Cunningham endorsed the practice because 'the potash and mucilaginous juices in the herbs and saliva neutralize or blunt the acrimony of the poison'.[8] Likewise, in 1859 Tasmanian surgeon (Edward) Swarbreck Hall recalled the 'fresh ashes of a particular plant being used as a specific for snake bites'.[9]

Of note amongst folk remedies was the insistence upon topical application. Whether employing local herbs or processed commodities such as tobacco juice, baking soda, turpentine or olive oil, vernacular treatments were generally rubbed in. Colonists were hardly reluctant to imbibe medicaments: by the 1820s Sydney offered a sound market for proprietary medicines such as the notorious Godfrey's Cordial.[10] When it came to snakebite, however, popular demand favoured external agents. Moreover, the quest for an effective antidote demanded *demonstrable* proof.

The persistent dismissal of Aboriginal knowledge

Intuitively, the most immediate source for such performances should have been the continent's Indigenous people. But the invaders – especially doctors – were fickle adopters of Aboriginal knowledge.[11] In early New South Wales, a snakebitten soldier gave 'all he was possessed of' – £5 – to the 'black physician' who pronounced a cure after applying a bark ligature, cutting the wound and sucking out the contaminated blood.[12] Nevertheless, it was a vast exaggeration to assert – as surgeon James Murray did in 1869 – that in the early years of settlement, 'thousands of valuable lives' had been 'undoubtedly saved by the simple remedies of the "savage"'.[13]

Lamentably, the dearth of Aboriginal accounts necessitates rendering Indigenous practices largely through settlers' descriptions – or speculation. Whilst paleopathologist Stephen Webb suggests that snakes posed a perpetual natural hazard, Indigenous historian Murray Johnson claims that 'the skilled bushcraft of Aboriginal Australians ensured that snakebite was an uncommon occurrence'.[14] We must furthermore be wary of conflating extraordinarily diverse Indigenous healing practices into an imaginary 'medical' unity spanning the entire continent.

This very variety mitigated against widespread settler embrace of Aboriginal remedies. In 1840, for instance, David Ballow – Colonial Assistant Surgeon at Moreton Bay – noted that an Indigenous man bitten by a snake first shrugged off the event, then fatalistically accepted his impending demise.[15] Such responses were distinct from nihilistic north-western Queensland cosmologies which saw in snakebite the implacable work of sorcery. Portents might also guide intervention. In Victoria's Western District, ethnographer James Dawson related in 1881 that when 'a person has been bitten by a snake, and has not been able to discern the species to which it belongs, he is made to look at the sun, and, if he sees an emu in it, the case is considered hopeless: he has seen his spectre, and must shortly die'.[16]

The modern term 'envenomation' is therefore freighted with biomedical implications inappropriate to many Aboriginal understandings. At the heart of this variability was the ontological status of the matter passing from snake to human, which was not necessarily 'venom'. It was believed in north-eastern New South Wales that bites introduced young snakes into the victim.[17] Elsewhere, venom merely provided a liquid conduit for the serpent's malevolent intentions. Other clans saw snakes – and venom – as agents of sorcery.

Nevertheless, it is astounding that John Burton Cleland – an assiduous compiler of historical health accounts – considered it 'doubtful whether before the coming of Europeans the aborigines had any idea that a poisonous snake injected venom, the effects of which might be alleviated by ligatures, rapid sucking, or scarification'.[18] Rather, almost all Indigenous approaches sought to extract or inactivate the material injected by the snake. Suction but not scarification was employed near the Swan River Colony in 1831, whilst another tribe squeezed the site to stimulate blood flow. In northern Australia – and possibly Tasmania – the bitten part would be irrigated by immersion under water. In Victoria, hot ashes were sometimes placed on the wound, whilst in several New South Wales and Tasmanian accounts, treatment comprised 'a kind of cauterisation, a hole being bored in the flesh near the wound and stuffed with fur, which was then singed'.[19] Informants frequently echoed Cunningham's 1827 summary from New South Wales that the 'native remedy is that practiced in all countries, namely, tying a tight ligature above the part, and scarifying and sucking the wound'.[20]

Indeed, Indigenous approaches were often marginalised precisely because they universalised the invaders' own customs. Whilst some settlers were disdainful of cutting, bleeding and sucking, such 'savage' techniques had been commonplace European responses to snakebite for millennia. Beyond the 1850s, reviews of Aboriginal healing tended increasingly towards dismissive antiquarianism.

Conversely, the most profound divergence between colonial and Aboriginal responses revolved around 'antidotes'. Indigenous people rarely employed external agents to counteract snakebite, even less commonly ingesting 'medicines'. Indeed, the only reported case in which an Aboriginal remedy was imbibed entailed veterinary rather than human patients.[21] Geography seems critical: 'bush medicines' across the continent's north may indicate historical syncretism with visiting Macassan traders, whose own preparations were suffused by contact with Chinese and Dutch medical systems.[22] One must therefore be cautious in presuming that reported Aboriginal remedies were 'timeless', or that their composition or use was faithfully conveyed to non-Indigenous observers.

Moreover, the truly divisive epistemological break centred around the colonisers' recourse to 'antidotes' and the means by which their efficacy was demonstrated. Animals proved central to this imperative. Indeed, goannas (*Varanidae* species) occupied an enduring place in the colonial animal matrix precisely because these large lizards attacked and killed snakes. 'A fight once witnessed can never be forgotten', declared Sydney University's lecturer in materia medica, John MacPherson.[23] As lampooned in 'Johnson's Antidote', it was widely believed that their imperviousness to envenomation could be attributed to, or bolstered by, consumption of a local plant.

Although many herbal remedies were vindicated by reference to analogous botanicals in India, the Philippines and the Americas, not all curative beliefs were so readily transplanted. Emerging from India by the mid-1600s, herbal, charcoal or bezoar-based 'snake stones' reputed to draw poison from a wound remained highly prized from Mexico to Cape Town until the end of the nineteenth century. Yet, having passed from European medical fashion, they barely figured in antipodean medical discourse, despite their reputed potency in curing human and animal patients alike.[24]

This indifference provides an intriguing counterpoint to the escalating circulation of putative therapeutics across colonial circumstances. It speaks, in the terminology of Arjun Appadurai, to the 'commodity context' by which things-in-motion accrue value within specific social and economic arenas.[25] In examining the transition of radium from an extraordinarily expensive scientific phenomenon to a constituent of toothpaste, for instance, Maria Rentetzi suggests that 'trafficking materials' accrue 'multiple identities, not because they are shared between different worlds but because they are transferred across them'.[26] Reversing the anthropological gaze to elaborate how the 'gift economy' of science appropriated and created value from culturally sensitive brain tissue samples, Warwick Anderson adds that the 'aura' of prior associations remains a critical element sustaining this traverse across economies.[27]

Narratives of animal sagacity, conversely, remained strikingly universal, perhaps because Australian colonists delighted in the frisson that they, like Johnson, might thus discover a lucrative yet quotidian local remedy. As the Bengal Army's Surgeon Major documented in 1868, 'the natives of India believe that ... if the mungoose [*sic*] be free after a contest with a cobra ... it will scamper off in search of some (unknown!) herb, and, eating it, become poison-proof'.[28] In 1894 Rudyard Kipling still felt obliged to discredit this enduring trope in 'Rikki-Tikki-Tavi'. Snakebite antidotes founded upon the silent testimony of goannas likewise sustained a reliable customer base. As late as 1913 the New South Wales Microbiological Laboratory reluctantly agreed to test such remedies, echoing Paterson's parody by finding 'death apparently being hastened rather than retarded by their use'.[29]

Snakebite as spectacle: public vivisection in the Australian colonies

According to the limited historiography on vivisection in Australia, animal experimentation rarely occurred in the colonial era.[30] Yet invasive experiments upon living creatures were not merely conducted,

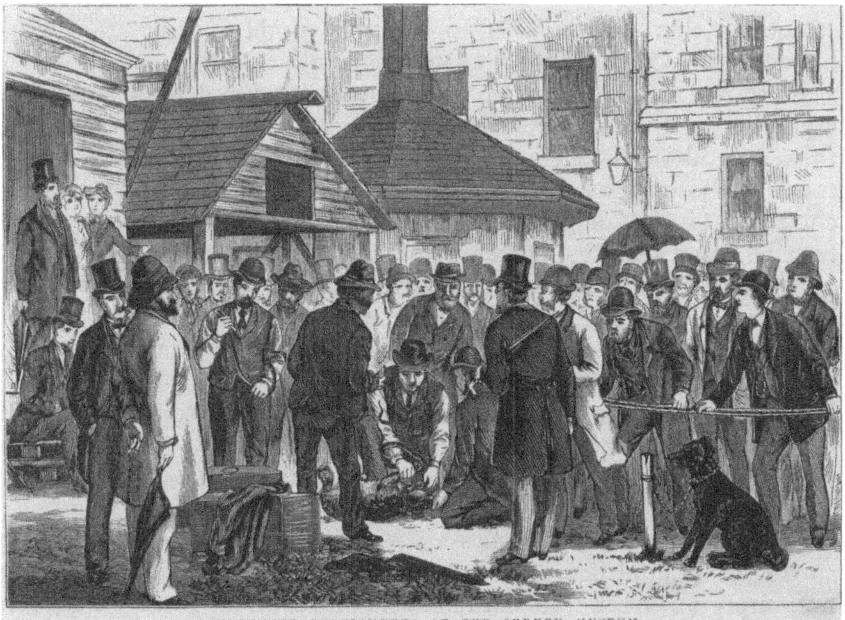

9 'Snake-bite experiments at the Sydney Museum', *Illustrated Sydney News and New South Wales Agriculturalist and Grazier*, 15 May 1880.

but widely accepted as models for human envenomation and its 'cure' across the colonies from the 1840s until World War I. Performed by lay spruikers and medical practitioners alike, such vivisections were widespread, profligate, frequently cruel and unashamedly public (Figure 9).

In his exploration of 'the ways that living beings have been transformed ... into living instruments and apparatus', science philosopher Rom Harré argues for setting aside ethical considerations in narrating how creatures have been integrated into the scientific 'instrumentarium'.[31] Yet the moral stakes for both human and non-human animals cannot be separated from their roles in experiments. This is not merely to reiterate William Coleman's assertion that 'understanding of life and organism and the suitability of one's means of investigation stand inseparable'.[32] Rather, the instrumentarium of vivisection extends beyond organic–inorganic dichotomies to incorporate affective, ethical and legislative considerations. Analysing animal experiments is as much a story of sensibility and sensitivity as it is of technologies and techniques.[33] To ignore such immaterial elements risks more than telling an incomplete tale; it perpetuates the objectivised narrative structures that have sought to expunge moral consideration from biomedical discourse since the late nineteenth century.

Until the 1850s, discursive use of 'vivisection' remained true to its etymology: the cutting or dissection of a living organism. Thenceforth, the term embraced wider meanings, largely through its growing deployment by those opposed to using animals for experiments in industrial chemistry, bacteriology, physiology, pharmacology or immunology. By the latter half of the century, 'vivisection' encompassed physical stimuli such as electricity, heat or trauma; the administration of chemicals, drugs and toxins; and the introduction of microorganisms to induce disease or produce therapeutic serums.[34] Concurrently, as its usage expanded amongst those promoting animal welfare or alternative medical epistemologies, reference to 'vivisection' subsided amongst experimentalists.

The very politicisation of the term – and its semantic transmogrifications across colonial arenas – has important historiographic implications. Because it was not necessarily actor parlance, particularly prior to the 1880s, the dearth of 'vivisection' in colonial discourse does not imply an absence of animal experimentation. British explorers intrigued by South American arrow poisons, for instance, tested the potency of curare upon oxen, horses and dogs.[35] The same substance intrigued early Brazilian physiologist João Baptista Lacerda, whose studies in animals extended to characterising local frog poisons and snake venoms.[36] Pratik Chakrabarti in particular has resurrected experimental 'beasts of burden' from Raj obscurantism, cloaked beneath a paternalistic moral opprobrium of Indian 'cruelties' towards brutes.[37]

Within the historiography of the Australian colonies such as Tasmania, for instance, Stefan Petrow has claimed that 'as no local experiments on animals apparently occurred, vivisection was not an issue' throughout the nineteenth century.[38] Yet that same colony hosted the first formal antipodean display of vivisection to study snakebite in 1850. Suggesting its significance, the demonstration was staged at Her Majesty's General Hospital in Hobarton (now Hobart) and documented in volume I of the *Papers and Proceedings of the Royal Society of Van Diemen's Land*. An early hub for both plebeian and exclusionary societies promoting scientific pursuits, the island colony was also foremost amongst the Australian settlements in seeking centralised oversight of medical practitioners and apothecaries via its hospital system.[39]

Instigated by government order, the experiments were overseen by a committee of military and medical officers, including James Agnew, later the colony's premier. Over 13–26 February 1850, layman Charles Underwood was encouraged to hurl dogs, cats and rabbits into a cage containing local diamond, whip, and brown or black snakes. When they did not bite voluntarily, he resorted to clasping each serpent's head, forcing the victim's nose or ear into its jaws. Underwood then applied his eponymous and popular snakebite antidote to approximately half of the bitten creatures.[40]

Whether or not Underwood's Antidote was dabbed onto the bite site, all three cats died. While no rabbit outcomes were recorded, the published subset comprising 25 of the 36 canine experiments suggested 28% mortality with antidote and 27% without. If these data permitted Agnew to later vindicate 'the unanimous conclusion that the application was valueless as an antidote', the full cohort was never analysed.[41] In fact, among animals bitten by black/brown snakes – the only species causing fatalities – 18% died following Underwood's Antidote, versus 31% without. Such *post-hoc* analyses are both simplistic and anachronistic, but the implications seem clear. Sanctioned by the colonial government and published for its scientific elite, the committee's cursory calculations underscored an official reluctance to dignify Underwood's claims. They did not, however, deride his methodology.

This acquiescence represented a critical juncture. Conducted within a formal institution, adjudicated by a learned committee and analysed by arithmetic, the mainland saw no equivalent snakebite series for another decade. But why did the island's cognoscenti allow this *amateur* to deploy his preferred heuristic tool – vivisection – rather than their own authoritative performances, particularly autopsy?[42]

Into the late 1840s, British practitioners were predominantly censorious of vivisection. Notoriously resistant to positivism and its implications for their lucratively individuated art of physic, from the 1830s Scottish- and English-trained clinicians nevertheless pursued increasingly localised approaches to medical investigation.[43] This spatial focusing – of patients into hospitals and maladies into lesions – intersected neatly with snakebite as a model for pinpointing the introduction of a noxious substance.

Critically, the shift towards vivisection appears to have been driven by Underwood himself. Peddling his snakebite remedy from October 1849 – immediately he was released from penal servitude – the Hobarton trial just four months later did little to stymy Underwood's trade.[44] Seamlessly conflating results from human and animal subjects, until his death in 1861 Underwood traversed towns, cities and colonies to demonstrate his snakebite remedy. Local serpents would be forced to bite a series of domesticated animals, and often the spruiker himself. Generally one victim received the antidote while another remained untreated.

If his performances proved erratic, Underwood's logic was consistent: the potency of snakebite and the efficacy of his curative could be demonstrated equally in animals or humans. Indeed, sales flyers asserted Underwood's readiness to 'submit his medicine to any test with rabbits, dogs, and other descriptions of animals, for the purpose of proving its efficacy in saving life'.[45] Lay audiences readily accepted such cross-species extrapolation. After he caused a Victorian 'yellow-bellied swamp snake' to bite a pigeon, a cat and two dogs in 1860, one canine survived after the antidote was 'instantly rubbed in', but the other did not. When Underwood 'offered to allow himself to be bitten, the audience would not permit the perilous experiment to be made'.[46]

Such *artificial* demonstrations of therapeutic efficacy saw vivisection serving as a spectacle across the Australian colonies.[47] Its popularity was paralleled by contemporaneous British fascination with mesmerism, another form of 'participatory theatre' skirting medical and scientific orthodoxy into the 1870s. Both transformed apparently neutral spaces into living laboratories, where – as Alison Winter has suggested – the crowd participated alongside the practitioner in generating and validating evidence.[48] Such displays questioned both the nature of proof required to constitute an 'experiment' and who was permitted to interpret its results. On trial were not simply competing authority claims, but deeper questions of epistemology within the very permeable boundaries of Victorian science.

Ritual sacrifices and institutionalised vivisection

This eager credulity encouraged the proliferation of both performances and practitioners. Chief amongst Underwood's challengers was another ex-convict, Joseph Shires. Emerging around 1860 in Tasmania (as Van Diemen's Land was renamed in 1856), he was more confident, more entrepreneurial and much longer-lived. Touting his own formula, Shires's antidote demonstrations interactively wove his audiences into the animal matrix. Capturing snakes from nearby bushland, he entreated locals to choose which would be employed. Inciting the crowd to submit their own domesticates for envenomation, punters thrust forth fowls, pet dogs and even 'a tough old pig ... kept for years and that had survived numerous encounters with venomous snakes'.[49] Shires likely made more money from these melodramatic performances than sales of his antidote, drawing crowds in streets, pubs, assembly rooms and finally – by the late 1860s – Melbourne's Canterbury Music Hall.

As with mesmerism in Britain, the ready transition of such performances from hotels to hospitals, thoroughfares to universities, showcased the insecurity of mid-century medical, scientific and legal authority. This instability necessitated not merely public demonstrations of 'proof', but of prevailing *systems* of proof. Such mobility – of materials, enactments and epistemological scaffolding – developed in parallel with the enormous popularity of international exhibitions as a means of disseminating the products and practitioners of Victorian science. 'Such events', notes Peter Hoffenberg, 'were essential to the generation, distribution, reception, and legitimacy of scientific knowledge and approaches, and the application of both to more general political, social, cultural and economic life'.[50] In each case, protagonists sought to accumulate social and financial capital within networks of verification, via what Appadurai refers to as 'tournaments of value'.[51]

Driven by the twinned commercial imperatives of entertainment and commoditisation, antidote shows foregrounded animal sacrifice as an intimate instantiation of a universal 'natural' phenomenon. What became increasingly important was not the validity of their method, but the verisimilitude of their claims. Touring Victoria together from 1860, Shires and Underwood drew the attention of magistrate George Clifford, who on 6 November 1861 convened a 'somewhat numerous gathering of scientific and medical men, as well as others interested in the subject of snakes and snake antidotes'. Also assembled at Melbourne's Richmond Police Barracks were 'troops of noisy curs, a quantity of fowls, a fine calf, and ... about a dozen snakes of all ages, sizes, and description'.[52] Nominally overseen by the Chairman of the Victorian Central Board of Health, William McCrea, Clifford decreed that pairs of animals should be bitten, with only one receiving the touted antidote. Despite offers made by Shires and Underwood, McCrea 'declined to permit any experiment to be made upon the men' – or, it seems, the fortunate calf.[53]

This tournament of value intricately interlaced the Victorian establishment into both the epistemology and the approbation of vivisection. With the bitten dogs removed under police custody until their demise or recovery, the serpents were conveyed to Melbourne University for identification by its Professor of Natural Science, Frederick McCoy. 'These experiments correspond very closely with those obtained in India and America', applauded the *Medical Record of Australia*, affirming that quotidian antipodean practices were beginning to intersect with the slow ascent of scientific vivisection across the Imperial west.[54]

Vipers, venom and vivisection

Until the early nineteenth century, extrapolating biological homologies from animals to humans remained both anatomically and theologically contentious. Usurping theist, deist or humanist rubrics, Jeremy Bentham's insistence on considering whether animals could suffer – rather than whether they possessed rational souls – provided opponents of vivisection with a more theriocentric ethic.[55] Likewise challenging natural history – dominated by morphology and thus by visual analogies between organisms – the vital difference distinguishing the emergent field of physiology was its elaboration of invisible internal characteristics and systems. Its mission, as Michel Foucault and Robert Frank have argued, was to elucidate the interior milieu and render the unity of unseen functional attributes knowable.[56]

Yet into the 1850s, there was no certainty that physiology would be dominated by experimentation. It was, as Coleman argues, 'long a science in search of a method'.[57] In England, John Hunter's influential vitalist schema held that the 'animal oeconomy' could be reduced to autonomous anatomical units linked by their ability to stimulate the 'living principle'. His conception of pathology was also critical in promulgating a physiological – as opposed to ontological – definition of illness. Hunter contended that the expression of disease was bounded by the functional possibilities of bodily structures, rather than determined by the properties of exogenous 'morbific' agents such as venoms.[58]

Nevertheless, both the mode and material of early physiology were shaped primarily by French practitioners under increasingly controlled environmental conditions. In his seminal *Formulary for the Preparation and Use of Many New Remedies* (1821), François Magendie affirmed the value of vivisection in claiming that 'medicines and poisons act in the same manner on man as on animals'.[59] From the 1850s, this new epistemology was exemplified and codified by Magendie's pupil, Claude Bernard. Propounding a theory of vital activity, in which biological processes were governed by a harmonious *milieu intérieur*, Bernard's highly influential *An Introduction to the Study of Experimental Medicine* (1865) extolled poisons as precise instruments for dissecting physiological processes, analogous to a scalpel localising anatomical features or pathological lesions.[60]

'It was Bernard, not Darwin, who provided a new system by which nature should be examined and controlled', proposes Carol Lansbury. 'Darwin changed what men believed, Bernard what they did.'[61] Although the chronological conjunction between Bernard, Charles Darwin's *On the Origin of Species* (1859) and the rise of vivisection appears patent, the moral impact of Darwinism was not straightforward. Animal activist Richard Ryder asserts that its 'central message, that the species are related through evolution, was not widely recognised as being of ethical importance in this context until the 1970s'.[62]

Furthermore, until the 1860s the scientific study of snakebite remained a very sparse field. Felice Fontana's landmark monograph – *Treatise on the Venom of the Viper* – had appeared in English as the First Fleet sailed for New South Wales in 1787. Chair of Physics at the University of Pisa, Fontana established the epistemological basis of toxinology by 'making experiments, decisive by their number, variety, and simplicity'.[63] He reported killing 3000 vipers and 4000 other animals which, asserts pharmacology historian Melvin Earles, comprised 'the most extensive series of experiments performed in the eighteenth century with the object of observing the effect of a single substance on living animals'.[64] Indeed, such extravagance with life remained rare until the close of the nineteenth century. Repeatedly insisting abhorrence at both the vast scale and individual suffering of his animal subjects, Fontana's qualms rarely stayed his hand. His antidote studies proved inconclusive but ultimately unfavourable, demonstrating that topically applied 'fluid volatile alkali' (ammonia) rarely preserved life, while in some animals it seemed to 'strengthen and reinforce the disease'.[65]

Fontana's exhaustive treatise and its nihilistic conclusions cast long shadows – both logistic and heuristic – over the subsequent century. Although rarely referenced in the Australian colonies, Fontana's British contemporary in India, Patrick Russell, cited his treatise but largely eschewed animal experiments.[66] The same pattern remained true until the 1860s, when Philadelphia physician Silas Weir Mitchell remarked that since 'the days of Fontana ... no researches of any moment had added to our knowledge of the poison of serpents'.[67] According to Mitchell's biographer, Nancy Cervetti, his own vivisections to study venoms represented 'the beginning of experimental medicine in the US'.[68]

Commencing in 1860, these studies were distinguished by Mitchell's commitment to the emerging ethos of continental physiology. Tutored by Bernard but ostensibly eschewing Fontana's largesse, by 1868 Mitchell had nevertheless killed hundreds of animals to explore rattlesnake venom.[69] Prompted by a reputedly 'infallible' Texan snakebite remedy, his first antidote series sacrificed merely a rabbit, 13 pigeons and 27 dogs. Jutta Schickore suggests that this parsimony was not primarily ethical, but epistemological. Accepting animal variability as an unavoidable consequence of vivisection, by constraining the number of experiments and reporting only 'representative' outcomes, Mitchell emphasised the priority of method over the mass of results.[70]

Published on the cusp of the Civil War, Mitchell's oeuvre established him as the Victorian heir to Fontana, the vivisector par excellence.[71] Yet he remained acutely aware of growing sensibilities towards inflicting pain upon living creatures, rationalising in 1868 that his experiments entailed 'a large expenditure of the lives of birds, dogs and rabbits, for which I am responsible to my own conscience, and to the Maker'. Apologising for eschewing chloroform because it might add 'new and obscuring elements', he claimed that 'the torture inflicted has been used with all possible thoughtfulness'.[72]

Sovereign remedies: evaluating animal evidence

Influential as Mitchell's work became, it formed just one bloodline coursing through the Australian colonies to build homologies between humans and animals. Recalling an 1860 performance by Charles Underwood, high-school headmaster George Metcalfe later recounted that 'People always doubted, and pondered thus: Was the snake venomous? Had its fangs been broken out? Was the antidote efficacious?'[73] When Underwood died in Melbourne on 27 December 1861 – attributed to 'the bite of a snake after the application of his own antidote' – magistrate George Clifford remarked, 'I have seen many experiments tried to test it, both publicly and privately ... [but] I never saw Underwood bitten by a snake which had killed any animal.'[74]

The critical element was the slippage between human and animal: the homology held. Clifford himself unwittingly afforded Underwood credence by admitting that he 'never recovered a single animal with his antidote'; one wonders whether these attempts were vivisectional or veterinary.[75] Indeed, even in the 1850s settlers proved increasingly willing to employ lay antidotes to treat their own snakebitten domesticates – especially dogs and horses. Despite their unstable commercial fortunes, the desire for universal antidotes – guaranteed by local consensus and purveyed by itinerant pedlars – fed into the sense of communitas and shared credulity generated by snakebite shows.

Indeed, both the composition and application of these remedies remained subordinate to their visible proof via animal experiment. Unlike the often-addictive cordials, tonics and elixirs forming the staple of 'quack' medicine, phials of Shires's Antidote bore a label directing the user to 'apply 10 drops to the par[t] bitten, and rub it into the blood. Caution – Poison'. Underwood remained a careless consumer of his own nostrum, occasionally forgetting to apply it at all. Moreover, however much they cut, bled or sucked the wound, settlers never introduced snakebite remedies into the bite site, nor were they ever swallowed.

This reticence to countenance internal use suggests numerous corollaries. Compared with observing goannas swallowing herbs, experimental proof of remedies in reluctant animal victims was simpler when antidotes were applied externally. Furthermore, vomiting was often the first response to snakebite, especially in dogs; perhaps the mode of application followed the mode of proof, rather than vice versa. Moreover, there was little suggestion that lay antidotes worsened the symptoms of snakebite. Indeed, the fact that these nostrums were not intended for consumption may explain their otherwise puzzling absence from Australia's controversial 1906–07 Royal Commission on Secret Drugs, Cures, and Foods.[76] Indeed, as late as 1934 the developers of the nation's first commercially produced antivenene found it necessary to discredit topically applied lay 'antidotes' – naturally, via vivisection.[77]

The challenge of the impregnable snake charmer

Through the nineteenth century, however, exchanges between laity and professionals were characterised as much by cooperation as competition. This convergence was both epistemological and aspirational: doctors sought not just to learn from antidote sellers, but to gain credibility from the association. In this endeavour they were not dissimilar to surgeons in India who, as Chakrabarti notes, regularly sourced knowledge and medicaments from 'local bazaars and practitioners'.[78] In Australia, any antagonistic undercurrents were predicated upon social rather than racial gradations, but most studies of snakebite remedies remained collaborative for several decades after 1860.

This is not to suggest that snakebite shows were universally lauded: in 1861, Underwood's untimely demise saw the inquest jury declaring that 'persons ought not to be allowed to exhibit poisonous snakes and to allow themselves or others to be bitten'.[79] Ironically, what ultimately drove Shires from his lucrative serpentine spectacles was the death of a police magistrate.

'It is not easy to conceive of a death more singular in its circumstances', opined London's *Medical Times and Gazette* in 1868, 'than that of Mr. William Henry Drummond.'[80] On 1 May, Drummond attended one of Shires's public seances, watching as the showman encouraged a tiger snake to bite himself and a fowl. The chicken died but Shires, applying his antidote, did not. Drummond remained sceptical and sought another demonstration. Not consenting to do so on stage, Shires accompanied the magistrate to a nearby hotel room. Taunting the showman, Drummond offered £1 and his own arm. After first protesting, Shires applied first a tiger snake, then his antidote. The reptile was decapitated for identification by Melbourne University's sole medical professor, George Halford, who was soon awakened by the arrival of both the serpent's head and the dying magistrate. The latter's demise – 'in spite of the enormous quantity of stimulants given' – provoked whispers of suicidal intent in Drummond, implications of medical laxity on Halford's behalf, accusations of manslaughter levelled at Shires, and renewed calls for the legislature to prohibit envenomation demonstrations. In the end, both pedlar and professor were exculpated by the court's acknowledgement that Shires's blood could tolerate the venom, 'just as vaccination renders one not susceptible of small pox'.[81]

If the Atlantic world showed little interest in acquired resistance until the 1880s, across the Empire the survival of snake charmers after serious bites mounted enduring challenges. Reassuring colleagues that showmen manipulated their serpents by removing fangs and draining glands of most of their venom, Halford's Australian rival for medical authority over snakebites – ophthalmologist Julius Berncastle – asserted in 1869 that 'you may take for granted that there is no immunity for any living person from the effects of the poison when fairly inoculated by it'.[82] Halford retorted that the rapid demise of snake handlers like Underwood proved that 'our snakes are as dangerous as those of India, and certainly quite as deadly as the Rattlesnake'.[83] In his 1870 monograph on Indian serpents, Bengal army surgeon Edward Nicholson considered Shires's case, believing previous exposure to sublethal bites sufficient to establish immunity. In his second edition of 1874 he elaborated that 'gradual inoculation of cobra-poison' might also explain the apparent immunity of Burmese snake charmers.[84]

The perpetual appeal of dying dogs

Despite Drummond's dramatic demise, lay demonstrations of snakebite antidotes remained lucrative, collaborative and authoritative. In a well-publicised 1880 experiment, conducted before 'a large number of scientific and other gentlemen', the grounds of Sydney's Australian Museum saw 'Several canine waifs and strays ... captured for the purpose of being handed over to the tender mercy of the snakes.'[85] After bites by serpents purchased for the Netherlands Government, Tamworth inventor Jean Baptiste administered his antidote to five dogs (Figure 9). Officiating was Edward Ramsay, the Museum's curator who claimed to have conducted many similar studies throughout the preceding five years; he may well have been the model for Paterson's 'scientific man'.

Trading upon the Museum's institutional credibility, these investigations remained a crowd spectacle. Staged not in a sequestered laboratory, but in a public courtyard, a rope was 'stretched across the enclosure at the back of the Museum to prevent crowding'. There was no doubt amongst this mob as to what was happening. When Ramsay incited a copperhead snake to bite, it proved 'a most severe one, drawing blood and eliciting loud cries from the dog', which later exhibited 'signs of having suffered severely from the poison injected into it'.[86] Baptiste's ineffectual remedy soon faded into obscurity, but what remained was the endorsement of similar antidotes by scientific institutions.

In utilising vivisection for this end, Sydney scientists were far from alone. At the Tasmanian Museum in Hobart, Curator Alex Morton found himself beset by antidote innovators over 1884–85, all requiring animal tests. Morton himself instigated another series of vivisections after witnessing the antidote demonstrations that charcoal burner 'Old Charley' performed upon himself.[87]

By the 1880s, however, the collaborative ethos became increasingly problematic. Repeating the Hobarton pattern set in 1850, Halford, Ramsay and Morton willingly observed as antidote vendors applied their own preparations. In 1877, however, doctors Tharp Girdlestone and William McCrea interrogated a touted antidote at the Melbourne Gaol (Figure 1). Having tested his remedy in animals, Queensland bushman James Hurst suggested that it should be applied to the wound after a tourniquet was tied. He therefore 'took exception' when Girdlestone and McCrea ignored these suggestions, instead using a hypodermic syringe to inject both the venom and Hurst's nostrum into a series of suffering hounds.[88] Unsurprisingly, their results proved unfavourable, as recent archaeological interpretation of the luckless animals' remains attests (Figure 10).[89]

A notable corollary was the diminution of human and serpentine agency. The Australian Museum experiments of 1880 maintained the direct snake-to-dog bite preferred by showmen and audiences. In the Melbourne Gaol, however, a diversity of devices was employed to capture and store snakes, milk their venom and inject it into the test animals (Figure 1). Such instrumentation and isolation of elements acted increasingly to neutralise lay experts and serpents alike. This formalised distancing accorded with the contemporaneous surge in zoo attendance and elite hunting which, proposes sociologist Adrian Franklin, enacted 'a ritual celebration of difference and superiority over animals'.[90]

Even into the *fin de siècle*, however, many of the conjunctions typifying plebeian antidote practice remained.[91] Early in 1897, the latest word in medical technology arrived in Melbourne: Albert Calmette's *Serum Antivenimeux*. A demonstration of this novel 'antivenene' assembled familiar elements: human and animal medicine, commercial and official interests, dogs and snakes, clinicians and showmen. It

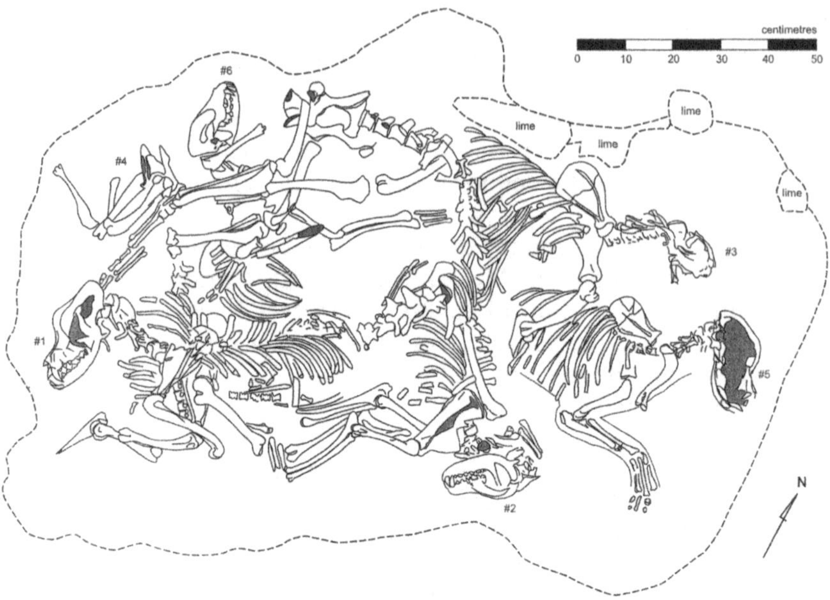

10 Geoff Hewitt, Gravesite of six dogs used in snakebite experiments within the Old Melbourne Gaol, 2002.

was conducted within the animal hospital of William Kendall, Principal of the Melbourne Veterinary College and Honorary Veterinary Surgeon of the Victorian Society for the Protection of Animals. Before several additional veterinary surgeons, members of the Victorian Board of Health and Calmette's Australian agents, the expensive serum was injected via hypodermic syringe into the shaved necks of dogs strapped to a surgical table. Yet applying tiger snakes directly to these constrained canines was 'Professor' William Davis, a well-known snake handler (Figure 30). After *Serum Antivenimeux* signally failed, Davis took a snakebite himself, dabbing on his own antidote and remaining 'as well as ever, with the exception of a very much swollen hand and wrist'.[92] The dogs, as usual, died.

Conclusion: the decline of public vivisection after 1880

Despite this seemingly ceaseless parade, the toll of experimental animals employed in public snakebite demonstrations declined after 1885. As snake showman John Cann has detailed, such performances relied increasingly upon self-experiment and stagecraft (Figure 11).[93] By 1903, conducting his final exhibition in rural Tasmania, 'Professor'

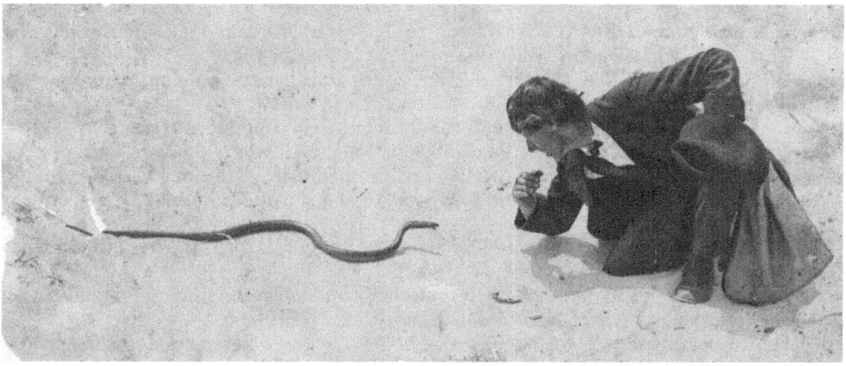

11 Frederick Fox and snake used for antidote experiments, *c.*1912.

Davis induced snakes to kill *only* three pigeons before accepting the bite that killed him. It is questionable whether he was even spruiking his antidote, let alone relying upon it.[94]

Ongoing public interest in such demonstrations indicated the enduring lay desire for an infallible snakebite remedy – and for performative proof of its efficacy in tournaments of value. The ascendance of self-experimentation suggests that whatever interest doctors displayed in constitutional immunity among those habituated to snakebite, it carried little popular credence. Perhaps the showmen's slide toward self-envenomation betrayed an acknowledgement of shifting sentiment – that killing animals was no longer an acceptable *public* practice. Yet few voices in Australia urged limiting animal experimentation until the 1920s.

The mid-Victorian era represented a transitional period in which, without sullying their clinical authority, medical practitioners permitted pedlars to demonstrate proprietary remedies both in themselves and in animal models. Reluctant to personally handle captive serpents, doctors were equally cautious in adopting public vivisection over 1840–80, although rarely for ethical reasons. Rather, there remained prodigious epistemological and political barriers to institutionalising vivisection as antipodean medical orthodoxy.

Notes

1 D. Graham Burnett, *Trying Leviathan: The Nineteenth-Century New York Court Case That Put the Whale on Trial and Challenged the Order of Nature* (Princeton: Princeton University Press, 2007), p. 8. See also Harriet Ritvo, *The Platypus and the Mermaid and Other Figments of the Classifying Imagination* (Cambridge, Mass.: Harvard University Press, 1998), pp. 51–68.

2 A.B. Paterson, 'Johnson's Antidote', in *The Man from Snowy River and Other Verses*, 4th edn (London: Macmillan and Co., 1896), p. 147.
3 C.J.S. Thompson, *The Mystery and Art of the Apothecary* (London: John Lane The Bodley Head, 1929), p. 61.
4 J.P. Griffin, 'Venetian treacle and the foundation of medicines regulation', *British Journal of Clinical Pharmacology*, 58:3 (2004), pp. 317–25.
5 Gael Phillips and John Pearn, 'Relict ancient medical practice in Australia', in John Pearn (ed.), *Health, History and Horizons* (Brisbane: Amphion Press, 1992), pp. 355, 361.
6 David L. Cowen and William H. Helfand, *Pharmacy: An Illustrated History* (New York: Harry N. Abrams, 1990), pp. 59–60.
7 Angeline Brasier, 'Prisoners' bodies: methods and advances in convict medicine in the transportation era', *Health and History*, 12:2 (2010), pp. 19–21.
8 Peter Cunningham, *Two Years in New South Wales*, 2nd edn, vol. I (Sydney: Angus and Robertson in association with the Royal Australian Historical Society, 1966), p. 165.
9 E. Swarbreck Hall, 'On snake bites', *Australian Medical Journal*, 4 (1859), p. 94.
10 Gregory Haines, *Pharmacy in Australia: The National Experience* (North Sydney: Australian Pharmaceutical Publishing Company, 1988), p. 21.
11 See, for instance, Frank Hansford-Miller, *Aboriginal and English Medicine in Swan River Colony in 1829* (Willetton: Abcado Publishers, 1990), p. 34; Luke Keogh, '*Duboisia pituri*: a natural history', *Historical Records of Australian Science*, 22:2 (2011), pp. 199–214.
12 [Untitled], *Hobart Town Gazette and Southern Reporter* (24 July 1819), p. 2.
13 J.P. Murray, 'Snake poisoning', *Australian Medical Gazette*, 1 (1869), p. 8.
14 Stephen Webb, *Palaeopathology of Aboriginal Australians: Health and Disease Across a Hunter-Gatherer Continent* (Cambridge: Cambridge University Press, 1995), p. 38; Murray Johnson, 'Fangs and faith: the search for an effective antidote against snake envenomation in Australia', *Journal of the Royal Australian Historical Society*, 95:2 (2009), p. 312.
15 D.W. Ballow, 'Caution to new-comers – death from the bite of a snake', *Sydney Gazette and New South Wales Advertiser* (9 April 1840), p. 2.
16 James Dawson, *Australian Aborigines: The Languages and Customs of Several Tribes of Aborigines in the Western District of Victoria, Australia* (Melbourne: George Robertson, 1881), p. 96.
17 Jeanette Covacevich, 'Phangs and physic: 40,000 years of risky business', in John Pearn and Mervyn Cobcroft (eds), *Fevers and Frontiers* (Brisbane: Department of Child Health, University of Queensland, 1990), p. 67.
18 J.B. Cleland, 'Aborigines: diseases and medicines', in *Australian Encyclopaedia*, 2nd edn, vol. 1 (Sydney: Angus & Robertson, 1958), p. 83.
19 G. Heuze Hogg, 'On the medicine of the Tasmanian aboriginals', in Gregory Sprott (ed.), *Intercolonial Medical Congress of Australasia. Transactions of the Sixth Session, Held in Hobart, Tasmania, February, 1902* (Hobart: John Vail, 1903), p. 176.
20 Cunningham, *Two Years in New South Wales*, p. 165.
21 J.H. Maiden, 'A reputed antidote to snake-bite', *Agricultural Gazette of New South Wales*, 5:7 (1894), p. 473.
22 Graham Connah, *The Archaeology of Australia's History* (Cambridge: Cambridge University Press, 1993), pp. 11–12; E.V. Lassak and T. McCarthy, *Australian Medicinal Plants* (North Ryde: Methuen, 1983), pp. 175–6.
23 John MacPherson, 'The treatment of snake-bite', *Australasian Nurses Journal*, 24 (1926), p. 56.
24 Martha Baldwin, 'The snakestone experiments: an early modern medical debate', *Isis*, 86:3 (1995), pp. 416–18.
25 Arjun Appadurai, 'Introduction: commodities and the politics of value', in Arjun Appadurai (ed.), *The Social Life of Things: Commodities in Cultural Perspective* (Cambridge: Cambridge University Press, 1986), p. 15.

26 Maria Rentetzi, *Trafficking Materials and Gendered Experimental Practices: Radium Research in Early 20th Century Vienna* (New York: Columbia University Press, 2007), p. 2.
27 Warwick Anderson, *The Collectors of Lost Souls: Turning Kuru Scientists into Whitemen* (Baltimore: Johns Hopkins University Press, 2008), pp. 133–4.
28 Charles R. Francis, 'On the action of cobra poison', *Indian Medical Gazette*, 3 (1868), p. 73.
29 J.B. Cleland, 'Alleged snake-bite remedies', in *Report of the Director-General of Public Health New South Wales, for the Year Ended 31st December, 1913* (Sydney: Government Printer, 1915), p. 250.
30 See for instance Jennifer MacCulloch, 'Creatures of culture: the animal protection and preservation movements in Sydney, 1880–1930' (PhD thesis, University of Sydney, 1993), pp. 79–88, 104; Philip Jamieson, 'Animal welfare: a movement in transition', in Suzanne Corcoran (ed.), *Law and History in Australia: A Collection of Papers Presented at the 1989 Law and History Conference* (Adelaide: Adelaide Law Review Association, 1991), pp. 27–9; Philip Jamieson, 'Duty and the beast: the movement in reform of animal welfare law', *University of Queensland Law Journal*, 16:2 (1991), pp. 239–49; K.D. Baker, 'Vivisection debate in nineteenth century Great Britain: a muted echo in colonial and early post-colonial Australia', *Australian Veterinary Journal*, 76:10 (1998), pp. 687–8.
31 Rom Harré, *Pavlov's Dog and Schrödinger's Cat: Scenes from the Living Laboratory* (Oxford: Oxford University Press, 2009), p. 2.
32 William Coleman, *Biology in the Nineteenth Century: Problems of Form, Function, and Transformation* (Cambridge: Cambridge University Press, 1985), p. 144.
33 Rob Boddice, 'Vivisecting Major: a Victorian gentleman scientist defends animal experimentation, 1876–1885', *Isis*, 102:2 (2011), p. 215.
34 Andreas-Holger Maehle and Ulrich Tröhler, 'Animal experimentation from antiquity to the end of the eighteenth century: attitudes and arguments', in Nicolaas Rupke (ed.), *Vivisection in Historical Perspective* (London: Croom Helm, 1987), p. 14.
35 Daniel John Hoffman, 'Fatal attractions: curare-based arrow poisons, from medical innovation to lethal injection' (PhD thesis, University of California, 2009), pp. 61–2.
36 Ana Carolina Vimieiro Gomes, '"Too good to be true": the controversy over the use of permanganate of potash as an antidote to snake poison and the circulation of Brazilian physiology in the nineteenth century', *Bulletin of the History of Medicine*, 86:2 (2012), pp. 158–62.
37 Pratik Chakrabarti, 'Beasts of burden: animals and laboratory research in colonial India', *History of Science*, 48:2 (2010), pp. 125–51.
38 Stefan Petrow, 'Civilizing mission: animal protection in Hobart 1878–1914', *Britain and the World*, 5:1 (2012), p. 79.
39 Colin Finney, *Paradise Revealed: Natural History in Nineteenth-Century Australia* (Melbourne: Museum of Victoria, 1993), pp. 33–62.
40 'Proceedings for July 1850', *Papers and Proceedings of the Royal Society of Van Diemen's Land*, 1:3 (1851), pp. 286–7.
41 J.W. Agnew, 'Notes on the poison of venomous snakes', *Papers and Proceedings of the Royal Society of Tasmania* (1864), p. 11.
42 See Helen MacDonald, 'A scandalous act: regulating anatomy in a British settler colony, Tasmania 1869', *Social History of Medicine*, 20:1 (2007), pp. 42–3.
43 W.F. Bynum, *Science and the Practice of Medicine in the Nineteenth Century* (Cambridge: Cambridge University Press, 1994), pp. 42–3, 49–50.
44 Maree Ring, 'Charles Underwood and his snake bite antidote', *Tasmanian Historical Research Association Papers and Proceedings*, 43:3 (1996), pp. 132–3.
45 W.E.L.H. Crowther, 'Mr. Charles Underwood and his antidote, with some observations on snake bite in Tasmania', *Medical Journal of Australia*, 1 (1956), p. 89.
46 'The disputed question of the efficacy of "snake antidotes"', *Australian Medical Journal*, 5 (1860), p. 240.

47 Peter Hobbins, 'Spectacular serpents: snakebite in colonial Australia', in Jacqueline Healy and Kenneth D. Winkel (eds), *Venom: Fear, Fascination and Discovery* (Melbourne: Medical History Museum, University of Melbourne, 2013), pp. 37–46.
48 Alison Winter, *Mesmerized: Powers of Mind in Victorian Britain* (Chicago: University of Chicago Press, 1998), p. 11.
49 John Cann, *Snakes Alive! Snake Experts & Antidote Sellers of Australia* (Kenthurst: Kangaroo Press, 1986), pp. 24–5.
50 Peter H. Hoffenberg, '"A science of our own": nineteenth century exhibitions, Australians and the history of science', in Brett M. Bennett and Joseph M. Hodge (eds), *Science and Empire: Knowledge and Networks of Science across the British Empire, 1800–1970* (Basingstoke: Palgrave Macmillan, 2011), p. 118.
51 Appadurai, 'Introduction', p. 21.
52 'Snake poison and its antidotes', *Argus* (8 November 1861), p. 3.
53 W. McCrea, 'Snake poison and its antidotes', *Argus* (12 November 1861), p. 5.
54 'Snake bites and their treatment', *Medical Record of Australia*, 1 (1861), p. 137.
55 Maehle and Tröhler, 'Animal experimentation from antiquity to the end of the eighteenth century', pp. 37–9; James Turner, *Reckoning with the Beast: Animals, Pain and Humanity in the Victorian Mind* (Baltimore: Johns Hopkins University Press, 1980), pp. 23–4.
56 See Michel Foucault, 'On the archaeology of the sciences: response to the Epistemology Circle', in James D. Faubion (ed.), *Aesthetics: Essential Works of Foucault 1954–1984*, vol. 2 (London: Penguin Books, 1998), pp. 314–15; Robert G. Frank, 'The telltale heart: physiological instruments, graphic methods, and clinical hopes 1854–1914', in William Coleman and Frederic L. Holmes (eds), *The Investigative Enterprise: Experimental Physiology in Nineteenth-Century Medicine* (Berkeley: University of California Press, 1988), pp. 211–90.
57 Coleman, *Biology in the Nineteenth Century*, p. 144.
58 Stephen J. Cross, 'John Hunter, the animal oeconomy, and late eighteenth-century physiological discourse', in William Coleman and Camille Limoges (eds), *Studies in History of Biology* (Baltimore: Johns Hopkins University Press, 1981), pp. 38–54.
59 François Magendie, *Formulary for the Preparation and Employment of Several New Remedies*, 6th edn, trans., Joseph Houlton (London: T. and G. Underwood, 1829), p. vii.
60 William Coleman, 'The cognitive basis of the discipline: Claude Bernard on physiology', *Isis*, 76:1 (1985), pp. 54–6.
61 Coral Lansbury, *The Old Brown Dog: Women, Workers, and Vivisection in Edwardian England* (Madison: University of Wisconsin Press, 1985), p. 155.
62 Richard D. Ryder, *Animal Revolution: Changing Attitudes towards Speciesism*, revised edn (Oxford: Berg, 2000), p. 61.
63 Felice Fontana, *Treatise On the Venom of the Viper; On the American Poisons; and On the Cherry Laurel, and Some Other Vegetable Poisons* (London: J. Murray, 1787), pp. 123–5.
64 M.P. Earles, 'The experimental investigation of viper venom by Felice Fontana (1730–1805)', *Annals of Science*, 16:4 (1960), pp. 255–6.
65 Fontana, *Treatise On the Venom of the Viper*, p. 152.
66 Barbara J. Hawgood, 'The life and viper of Dr Patrick Russell MD FRS (1727–1805): physician and naturalist', *Toxicon*, 32:11 (1994), p. 1302.
67 S.W. Mitchell, 'Experimental contributions to the toxicology of rattle-snake venom', *New York Medical Journal*, 6:4 (1868), p. 289.
68 Nancy Cervetti, 'S. Weir Mitchell and his snakes: unraveling the "united web and woof of popular and scientific beliefs"', *Journal of Medical Humanities*, 28:3 (2007), p. 120.
69 S. Weir Mitchell, 'On the treatment of rattlesnake bites, with experimental criticisms upon the various remedies now in use', *North American Medico-chirurgical Review*, 5:2 (1861), p. 271.
70 Jutta Schickore, 'Scientists' methods accounts: S. Weir Mitchell's research on

the venom of poisonous snakes', in Seymour Mauskopf and Tad Schmaltz (eds), *Integrating History and Philosophy of Science: Problems and Prospects* (Dordrecht: Springer, 2011), pp. 147, 154–7.

71 W. Bruce Fye, 'S. Weir Mitchell, Philadelphia's "lost" physiologist', *Bulletin of the History of Medicine*, 57 (1983), pp. 190–1.

72 Mitchell, 'Experimental contributions to the toxicology of rattle-snake venom', p. 290.

73 G. Metcalfe, *Australian Zoology* (Sydney: E.W. Cole, 1895), p. 46.

74 'Death from a snake-bite. Adjourned inquest on the body of Underwood', *Argus* (1 January 1862), p. 6.

75 'The disputed question of the efficacy of "snake antidotes"', p. 11.

76 See Lynette Finch, 'Soothing syrups and teething powders: regulating proprietary drugs in Australia, 1860–1910', *Medical History*, 43:1 (1999), pp. 89–93.

77 Peter G. Hobbins, 'Serpentine science: Charles Kellaway and the fluctuating fortunes of venom research in interwar Australia', *Historical Records of Australian Science*, 21:1 (2010), pp. 10–11.

78 Pratik Chakrabarti, *Materials and Medicine: Trade, Conquest and Therapeutics in the Eighteenth Century* (Manchester: Manchester University Press, 2010), p. 184.

79 Ring, 'Charles Underwood and his snake bite antidote', p. 136.

80 'The fatal snake-bite at Melbourne', *Medical Times and Gazette*, 2 (new series 37) (1868), p. 99.

81 'Fatal experiment with a snake', *Illustrated Australian News for Home Readers* (16 May 1868), p. 7.

82 Dr Berncastle, 'The treatment of snake-bites', *Australian Medical Gazette*, 1 (1869), p. 34.

83 George B. Halford, 'The treatment of snake-bite in Victoria', *Australian Medical Journal*, 15 (1870), p. 171.

84 Edward Nicholson, *Indian Snakes. An Elementary Treatise on Ophiology with a Descriptive Catalogue of the Snakes Found in India and the Adjoining Countries*, 2nd edn (Madras: Higginbotham and Co., 1874), p. 148.

85 'A snake-bite antidote', *Illustrated Sydney News* (15 May 1880), p. 7. Unfortunately, no record of these experiments could be located in the Australian Museum archives.

86 *Ibid.*

87 Ring, 'Charles Underwood and his snake bite antidote', p. 139; Crowther, 'Mr. Charles Underwood and his antidote', p. 88.

88 'Sketches of snake-bite experiments in the Melbourne Gaol', *Australasian Sketcher with Pen and Pencil* (17 February 1877), p. 182.

89 R.L. Buckley, 'Six dogs: a saga of snakes, dogs and medical byways' (BA (Hons) thesis, La Trobe University, 2003), pp. 54–9, 76–80.

90 Adrian Franklin, *Animals and Modern Cultures: A Sociology of Human–Animal Relations in Modernity* (London: Sage, 1999), p. 30.

91 John Cann, *Historical Snakeys* (Rodeo: ECO Publishing, 2014), *passim*.

92 'Snakebite and antidote', *Queenslander* (20 February 1897), p. 421.

93 Cann, *Snakes Alive!* pp. 35–60.

94 'Snake charmer's end. Death of "Professor" Davis. Bitten by a tiger snake. The inquest', *Examiner* (5 May 1903), p. 6.

CHAPTER THREE

Ontological conjunctions: dogs, snakes, venoms and germs, 1840–68

Public demonstrations helped establish the dangerous *action* of snake venom through the mid-nineteenth century, but they provided little elucidation as to its *nature*. Was it animal, germinal or chemical?

This fundamental question proved ontological in two senses. First, venom provided an exemplar of an ontological agent of disease: a discrete entity causing a reproducible syndrome across diverse populations of victims.[1] If Pasteurian germ theory saw such an aetiological approach typify 'scientific medicine' over the latter half of the century, in the Australian colonies, experiments in domestic animals had helped establish venom as an autonomous agent long before 1860.

Second, characterising venom comprised an operation of historical ontology. Germ theory proved central to this process, as did its primary tool: the microscope. By agreeing on what they could or could not see, elite investigators defined what venom could or could not be. Moreover, to confirm their hypotheses regarding the nature of venom, medical scientists arranged specific conjunctions of instruments and creatures – particularly snakes and dogs. Although this reshuffling of the animal matrix drew heavily upon plebeian traditions, after 1868 the staging and interpretation of animal experimentation shifted steadily from the public gaze.

There was no inevitability about this process. Central to this chapter is a controversial incident: George Halford's germ theory of snake poisoning. Explaining its intercolonial demise certainly requires attention to what David Livingstone identifies as the 'diffusion tracks along which scientific ideas and their associated gadgetry migrate'.[2] But there was more to the fate of Halford's theorem than mobility; nor can it entirely be explained as a failed paradigm. While Thomas Kuhn attributed the success of paradigms largely to their ability to generate concordance between diverse communities of investigators, they are also underpinned by the acceptance of theories and instrumentation which inherently constrain the range of grounds for agreement.[3] These limitations govern what Ian Hacking articulates as historical ontology, 'the ways in which the possibilities for choice, and for being, arise in history'.[4]

In the colonial antipodes, there was no inherent nexus governing the fundamental nature of venom. Rather, it occurred at 'working surfaces' comprising intersections between animals, instruments, spaces and discourses, generating novel epistemological and ontological possibilities.[5] Such assemblages, argues Lorraine Daston, affirmed the collective empiricism by which 'expert observation discerns and stabilises scientific objects for a community of researchers'. Indeed, nineteenth-century microscopy exemplified the necessity for repeated observation and the role of trained observers in negotiating collective agreement about the very existence of new phenomena. Seeing something was not enough; it was the sense of immediate recognition – of shared gestalt – that stamped nascent ontologies 'with the imprimatur of the really real'.[6] When this recognition was withheld from practitioners on the margins of scientific communities, neither their authority nor their ontology were 'seen'.

The absence of invisible entities: venom to 1843

In the Australian colonies, despite a perennial fear of serpents (Figure 12), little was published regarding the nature of snake venom until the 1840s. The first speculations comprised reprinting an 1801 article by Bombay surgeon William Boag, who believed that venom acted chemically to deoxygenate the blood of its victims.[7] Concurring that blood formed its chief seat of mischief, in 1826 Sydney surgeon William Bland recommended cupping glasses to draw out the poison.[8] He decreed his clinical successes superior to the animal experiments recently performed by John Barry at the Royal Institute of France. Employing suction to remove the poisons of venomous and rabid creatures, Barry's vivisections proved influential in Europe, but not in the Australian colonies.[9] Despite the hecatombs of experimental animals sacrificed to study venom, noted Hermann Schlegel – the era's most influential herpetologist – its essence remained obscure. Beyond a measurable dose–response effect, its actions were shaped by the ambient temperature and the 'violent emotions' of both serpent and victim.[10]

Yet poisons could arguably have formed a centrepiece for antipodean natural philosophy. In 1835, James Apjohn – Professor of Chemistry at Ireland's Royal College of Surgeons – proposed that in spanning natural history, chemistry, pathology and physiology, the emergent field of toxicology required 'such an extensive acquaintance with

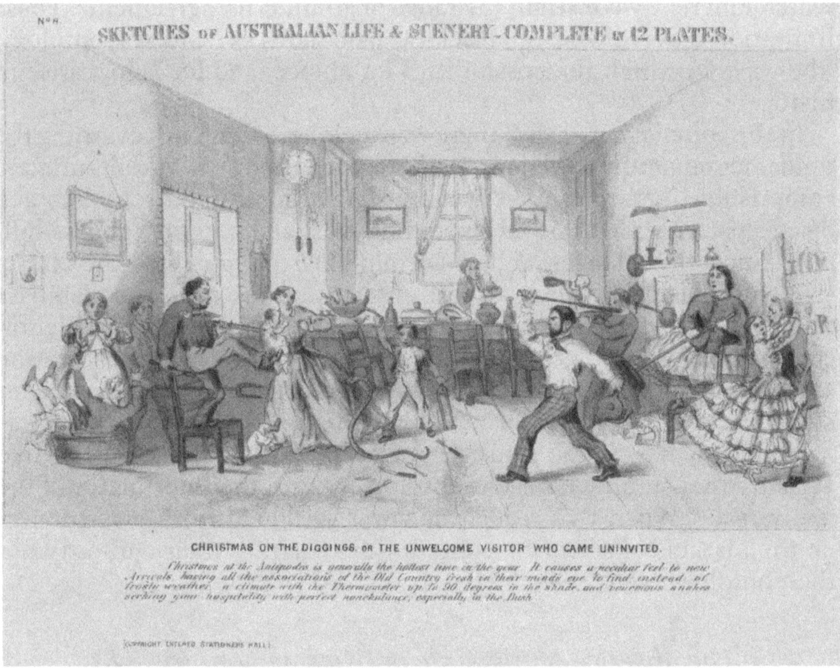

12 'Christmas on the diggings or the unwelcome visitor who came uninvited', *Sketches of Australian Life and Scenery Complete in 12 Plates* (London: Paul Jerrard & Son, *c.*1860).

many departments of natural knowledge as rarely falls to the lot of any individual'. Declaring the Indian cobra and American rattlesnake the deadliest known serpents, Apjohn admitted that toxicologists had not yet 'ascertained whether the poison of venomous reptiles acts by entering the blood, or is the result of nervous sympathy'.[11]

Australian enquiries remained episodic. 'In 1841', recalled government explorer and surveyor Clement Hodgkinson, 'the nature and effects of the poison of snakes had been little discussed'.[12] Bitten by 'a large black snake', his saviours included local Aborigines who sucked the bite site, and a former surgeon who opened the wound before applying nitric acid. This apparent neutralisation led Hodgkinson to query whether the poison was 'alkalescent', testing both black snake and death adder venom on blue litmus paper. The results suggested that two specific remedies were required to counteract snake bites: one for the acidic form causing pronounced local reactions, another for the more neutral variety with 'effects analogous to those of a depressing narcotic poison'.[13] Citing both human and canine fatalities, in 1845 he claimed for the death adder the most potent venom of any Australian snake, noting that its general paralytic action closely resembled that of Egyptian cobras, rather than the localised damage caused by American rattlesnake or European viper bites.[14] By 1847, even Bland acquiesced, detailing experiments conducted by his stepson, Henry Smeathman, who placed the thighs of young chickens within the mouths of dead serpents, causing a 'bite'. Venoms, Bland recapitulated, were capable of 'much derangement of the general health', but ventured no suggestion regarding their nature.[15]

Championing a comprehensive scheme of vivisection

Perhaps the most striking venom study in nineteenth-century Australia is a largely overlooked paper by Irish-born surgeon and later Premier of Tasmania, James Agnew. Published in 1846, it comprised the first systematic study of the dentition and venom glands of Australian ophidians. Agnew confirmed the potency of 'the clear, glairy, venomous fluid' by administering it with fatal results in several small animals. Appealing for experiments across the Australian colonies, he championed a comprehensive scheme of vivisection to characterise 'the comparative intensity of the poison in the different species, and how this may be modified by the season of the year and other circumstances'.[16]

Few responded. Observing that 'the serpents of this country had scarcely received the attention which their importance demands', over 1858–59 Alfred Roberts – honorary surgeon at the Sydney Infirmary and Dispensary – published a preliminary survey.[17] His intricate dissections and dental descriptions challenged the prevailing classification propounded by French zoologists André Marie Constant Duméril and Gabriel Bibron. Cleaving snakes into Innocua or harmless serpents, and Venenosa or poisonous snakes, their anthropocentric schema was one of 'no less than sixteen', Roberts noted.[18] As Harriet Ritvo remarks, 'the claim of human authority implicit in the notion of scientific taxonomy was more significant than the specific content of competing systems'.[19]

Reinforcing the endemic disputes between functionalists and structuralists across Victorian comparative anatomy and taxonomy, Roberts's alternative schema centralised the function of venom.[20] He argued that relying entirely upon structural criteria – à la Duméril and Bibron – rendered it 'impossible to define accurately the line of demarcation between a truly venomous and an equally innocent snake'.[21] His observations of the direct effects of snakebite – in cats, rats, mice, frogs and insects – saw Roberts emphasise the role performed by poison. Primarily designed to aid digesting prey, killing victims comprised its secondary function, its defensive use being merely tertiary.

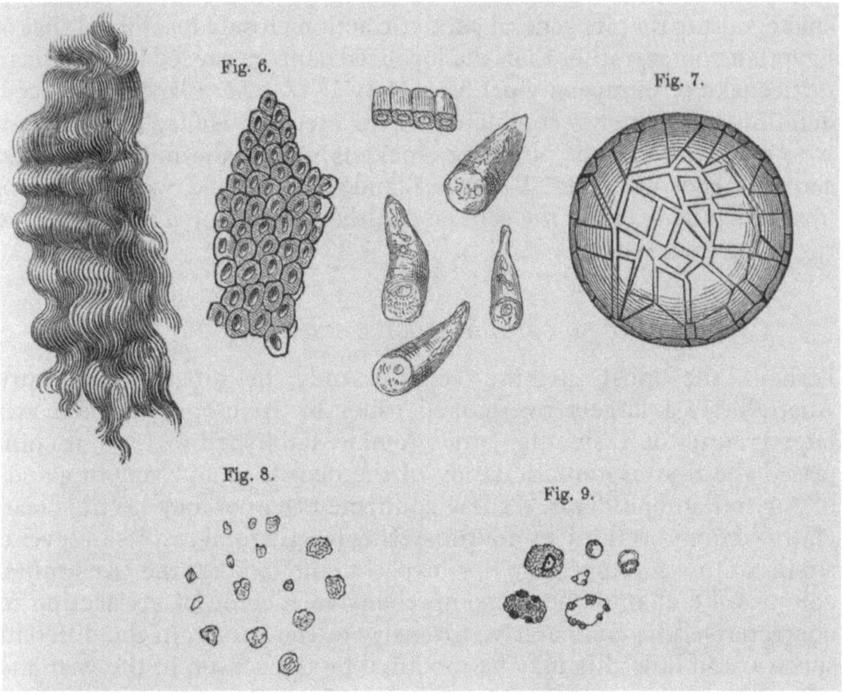

13 Alfred Roberts, 'On the structure and function of the poison apparatus in venomous serpents, with a description of some of the species found in Australia', *Sydney Magazine of Science and Art* (1859).

Of most interest, moreover, was Roberts's investigation of venom as an isolated entity (Figure 13). Microscopically, it displayed no visible markers of pathogenicity, beyond granular bodies which degraded when treated chemically with acetic acid. Attempting to discern the smallest functional unit embodying the potency of snake poison, Roberts – like many contemporaries – enlisted cellular pathology to determine the aetiological basis of a disease. By 1860, as Michael Worboys details, morbid processes hitherto regarded as purely chemical were coming to be seen as essentially vital.[22] Aware of Louis Pasteur's studies linking microorganisms to fermentation and putrefaction, Roberts dismissed this explanation, but remained rare amongst colonial doctors in suggesting that venom might in some manner be 'alive'.

Ontological ferment: venom in the early 1860s

By 1860, contrasts between divergent patterns of envenomation were increasingly being drawn between different regions of the world. In part this toxicological cosmopolitanism can be attributed to an index Imperial event: the 1852 death of a keeper at London Zoo following an Indian cobra bite. After its venom was studied via post-mortem examination, chemical tests and injection of the victim's blood into a mouse, pragmatic advice on snakebite management radiated forth from the Metropole to colonial practitioners.[23] Authoritative pronouncements continued henceforth to be broadcast by stalwart institutions such as the *Lancet* and the British Museum.[24]

But the thick-crossed diffusion tracks of mid-century science also connected continents without centralised mediation. As colonial animal encounters multiplied, documentation and speculation escalated, alongside the movement of serpents themselves. Developing from an ophidian Orientalism, after 1850 'snakes and snakebite mortalities dominated the official and popular discourse in British India', notes Pratik Chakrabarti.[25] Fluctuating between fieldwork and pharmacology, Calcutta-based studies sought to systematise knowledge and allay alarm across the principalities. Concurrently, considers Kay Anderson, an escalating commerce in zoological exchange saw cobras institutionalised among the 'staple creatures' which circuited the globe as embodied 'emblems of colonial mastery over the animal world'.[26] Private commerce was even more frenzied, with British 'wild beast merchants' selling snakes 'by the mile' – including cobras.[27]

As identified snake species proliferated, distinctions between specific toxicities and the overall 'virulence' of venoms followed suit.[28] To paraphrase Ernst Haeckel, ontology recapitulated phylogeny, prompting the deployment of technologies such as microscopy and analytical chemistry to enumerate the properties of individual venoms. In 1859 (Edward) Swarbreck Hall, an aspiring medical scientist in Tasmania, urged 'a chemical analysis of those terrible organic compounds' to discern what 'combination of elementary substances it is that gives the lethal properties to the snake poisons'.[29] Deducing from post-mortem examinations that venom both coagulated and deoxygenated the blood, Hall numbered among the few doctors who prepared detailed autopsy reports to discern the specific pathophysiology of snakebite.[30]

Such considerations foregrounded venom as an autonomous agent. In Sydney, Roberts was vexed by the observation – far from novel even in 1859 – that dehydrated venom retained its potency indefinitely. He confirmed this property via experiments in kittens who, whether administered fresh or reconstituted death adder venom, 'died within an hour, apparently in pain'.[31] Unable to discern any divine logic undergirding this enduring efficacy, he concluded that it must comprise a chemical agent created by vital processes. Roberts likewise puzzled over the *in vivo* effects of this 'animal fluid'. Was venom a general toxin disseminated via the circulatory system? Did it alternately effect a 'morbid change', such as fermentation, in the blood? Or did venom somehow completely extinguish 'vital power' in its victims?

If not the only means of answering such fundamental questions, living proofs became more prominent by the mid-1860s. Now elected Honorary Secretary of the Royal Society of Tasmania, James Agnew returned to snakebite in 1864. Pressing the contents of one dissected 'black snake' venom gland into the scarified leg of a young chicken, he forced the other gland down a second pullet's throat. Repeating the experiment in a brace of kittens, he declared his results 'so decisive, that I did not think it necessary further to repeat observations which would only necessitate pain and loss of life, without adding anything to the certainty or truth of the conclusions arrived at'.[32] Seemingly humane, his parsimony arose chiefly from the patent outcome of these vivisections: ingested venom was innocuous, absorbed venom deadly.

As with contemporary lay antidote demonstrations, this epistemological connection between animal data and human application appeared unproblematic. Moreover, Agnew's experiments betrayed an increasingly ontological conception of venom as an autonomous 'pathogen', rather than an indiscriminate chemical 'poison'. Indeed, in the 1860s snake venom arguably provided a more credible aetiological agent than microorganisms, for which causal links with clinical symptomatology remained far from proven.[33]

'A case of genuine hydrophobia in Hobart Town'

Serpents, however, were not the only beasts believed capable of generating and transmitting noxious substances via their bites. The zoonotic nature of rabies was recognised by the ancients, and seventeenth-century doctors maintained the Galenic belief that 'poyson is bred in Dogs when they are mad, which is very infectious'.[34] Medical texts consistently grouped the condition alongside animal venoms, but set rabies apart on account of its mammalian hosts, latency of onset and potential infectivity through chains of victims. By the turn of the nineteenth century, the saliva of rabid animals was rarely labelled 'venom', but its ontological status remained unstable. Well into the 1880s, laity and practitioners alike feared that ill breeding, inherent 'weakness' or insalubrious climate might spontaneously generate rabies in their canine companions, although its relationship to the analogous human condition of hydrophobia remained contentious.[35]

Until 1800, as James Boyce has elaborated, no canid had ever set paw on Tasmania, yet by 1830 swelling dog numbers saw the island's settlers enacting one of the world's first Dog Acts.[36] British attempts to contain unruly hounds likewise escalated over 1865–66, the 'years of general pestilence' marked in Britain by the fourth visitation of cholera, a devastating cattle plague and rising concern over rabies.[37] In the penumbra of such portents, a 'case of genuine hydrophobia in Hobart Town' was reported early in 1867. On 19 January a black 'half-bred spaniel bitch' became, according to local surgeon Thomas Smart, 'unusually vicious and quarrelsome ... frothing at the mouth, &c'.[38] It was soon found dead, but not before wounding other dogs and four human victims. Three appeared safe; not so nine-year-old Thomas Bowring, nipped on the lip.

After an initial recovery, Bowring began displaying agitation, headache and loss of appetite. This proceeded to vomiting, frequent urination and hypersalivation of 'viscid ropy mucus', which he clawed from his mouth with 'sounds resembling the barking of a dog'. Smart was more concerned by the boy's violent response to a cup of water, being 'instantaneously seized with a paroxysm of indescribable terror'.[39] By 17 February, Bowring was impulsive, unsteady and incoherent, attempting to bite both his own hand and his mother's shoulder. Shortly thereafter he died in her arms.

As scripted by Smart, Bowring's symptoms closely matched prevailing depictions of hydrophobia. Immediately alarmed, the surgeon consulted five respected colleagues, including Agnew and Hall. At the Health Committee of the Municipal Council of Hobart Town, all six concurred that 'this case was one of Rabies or Hydrophobia': its first report across any of the Australian colonies.[40]

If historical opinion remains divided as to whether this constituted a 'true' case, in 1867 the alarm was palpable.[41] Relaying a newspaper report that two 'rabid dogs' had died in convulsions at Hobart's military barracks, the *Australian Medical Journal* found 'no reason for doubting that hydrophobia has been acclimatized in the island colony'.[42] Hall reported another dog nipping a 'respectable' woman, adding that 'hydrophobia exists among dogs to a greater extent than the case of Bowring would lead one to suppose'.[43] The Health Committee immediately recommended a police round-up of unruly or unhealthy canines – primarily for extermination.

The sole dissenting voice was William Lodewyk Crowther, a Dutch-born surgeon and naturalist who – like Agnew – later served as Tasmanian Premier. Without visiting the patient, Crowther proposed that Bowring's symptoms suggested a more mundane condition: traumatic tetanus. The resultant acrimonious exchanges undermined the credibility of Tasmanian observers and, lacking further cases, the episode promptly withered.

Although Tasmanian clinicians might have utilised their geographical isolation as a unique opportunity to investigate the idiopathic emergence of rabies, neither Agnew nor Hall studied tissue or saliva samples from the suspect dog or its victims. Yet esteemed anatomist John Hunter had suggested as early as 1793 that saliva from a rabid dog could be inoculated into other canines; a decade later Georg Gottfried Zinke utilised this technique to establish the transmissibility of rabies.[44] Evidence from other colonised territories such as southern Africa concurrently bolstered and belittled climatological or topographical aetiologies. But the canine culprits, notes Karen Brown, remained identical.[45] If the persistent belief in spontaneous generation 'shifted moral responsibility from the infected dog to cruel human caretakers', as Ritvo proposes, contagionist hypotheses imputed culpability to the rabid animal.[46] However, as Pat Macwhirter details for other putatively zoonotic diseases in the 1860s, neither established clinical authority nor empirical observation were sufficient to confirm or reject contagionist postulates.[47]

A critical lacuna was the absence of instrumentation. On the mainland, microscopes legitimated contemporaneous claims by experimenting pastoralists that sheep scab was both transmitted by a parasitic mite and eradicable via chemical dipping.[48] But ontological transformations required more than magnification. As Bruno Latour argues, the critical technique for Pasteur's rabies studies was neither microscopy nor experimental inoculation. Rather, the labours of bacteriologists, their materials and microbes were all commandeered in the performative space of the laboratory to craft an entirely new entity: laboratory rabies.[49]

Indeed, Latour asserts, laboratories elide a fundamental epistemic contradiction in enabling both artificer and artefact to speak autonomously.[50] By translocating gestures, techniques and devices from the laboratory into the clinic and field, 'the reality of Pasteur's germ' was reified via 'an ever greater number of elements with which it [was] associated – machines, gestures, textbooks, institutions, taxonomies, theories'.[51] Hall and Agnew had employed analogous measures in conducting and communicating their snake venom studies, but failed to similarly manifest the *materiality* of hydrophobia.

By 1867 the concordance of clinicians proved insufficient to transport the 'reality' of Tasmanian rabies to the mainland, let alone Britain. The prevailing historical ontology of rabies – as an autonomous poison that could pass from animal to animal, and from animal to human – demanded material proof beyond mere testimony. Indeed, the 1860s represented a shifting landscape for exogenous 'germs' as *contagium viva*. Drawing together dogs, snakes, venoms and germs within a different matrix, a more productive 'choreography of truth' eventuated in Victoria just a few months later.[52]

Colonial curs and a Ceylonese cobra

The SS *Bombay* docked in Melbourne on 14 April 1867. Amongst the passengers filing off this intercolonial steamer was manure merchant, John Barton Burstall, who had boarded in Ceylon. Securing lodgings at Tankard's Temperance Hotel, Burstall invited fellow travellers to his bedroom. He had something to show them.

Removing the lid of a wicker basket, Burstall lifted out a languid cobra-di-capella, later demonstrating its docility by draping the serpent around his neck. Having wrenched out its fangs before leaving Ceylon, he remained unconcerned at the swelling where the snake had scratched his left hand, or when it again bit the same hand.[53] Shortly afterwards, however, fellow guest Francis Fielder 'remarked a peculiar sound in one of the bedrooms, something between a low whine and a moan, which he thought appeared to come from some human being'; another visitor 'suggested it was a dog'.[54]

Entering the bedroom, the two men found Burstall writhing in agony, grasping his swollen hand. Fielder applied a ligature, scarified the bite and washed it with brandy, forcing a measure down Burstall's gullet, 'which produced vomiting and for a time cleared his throat of a quantity of ropy, viscous slime'.[55] Local surgeon Thomas Fitzgerald found Burstall in a stupor, his speech incomprehensible and subject to frequent bouts of loose diarrhoea. Fitzgerald administered more brandy, followed by ammonia and strong coffee via a stomach pump, but to little avail. Burstall's pulse faded and he expired shortly after being conveyed to the Melbourne Hospital.

If details of John Burstall's demise were typical of nineteenth-century envenomation reports, the cobra's participation escalated the epistemological stakes. The transnational exchanges arising from this incident both encapsulated the universalising mission of 'modern' medical science whilst undercutting its claims to transcend locality and particularism. It also prefigured the global circulation of snakes, venoms and experimental data that generated profound ontological questions about 'the animal' in this rapidly Darwinising age.

One figure united and divided these networks: George Britton Halford (Figure 14). 'One of the most distinguished experimental physiologists of the day', in 1863 Oxford-trained Halford became Melbourne University's inaugural Professor of Anatomy, Physiology and Pathology – the first teaching professor of medicine in the antipodes.[56] Arriving with a sound reputation for physiological research

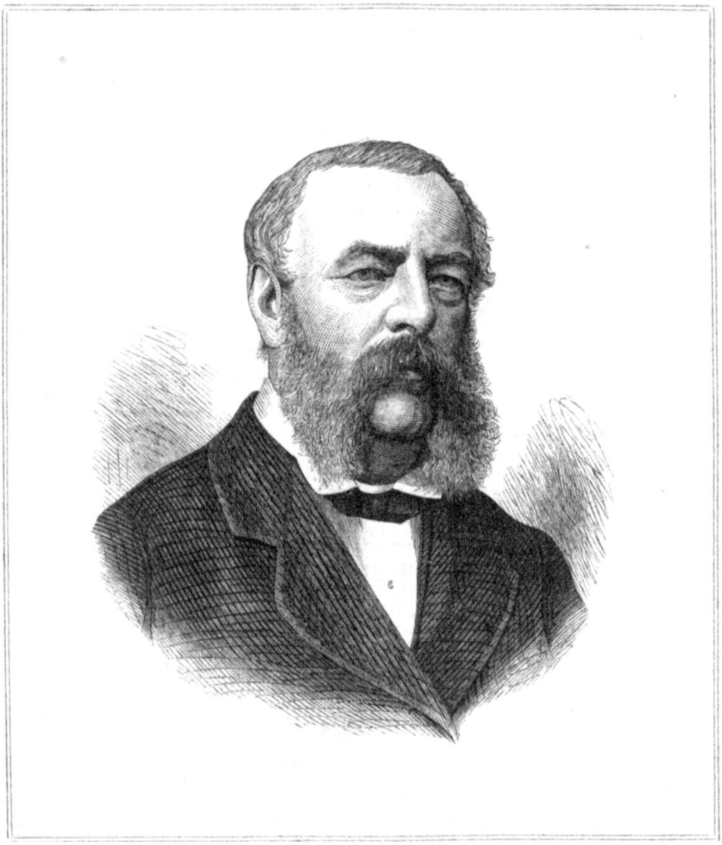

14 'Professor Halford, M.D., F.R.S.', *Leader* (Melbourne), 26 November 1881.

on human and animal hearts, function formed the heuristic centre of his medical pedagogy: his 'zealous spirit of investigation' reportedly encouraged colonial doctors to 'the honest pursuit of medical science'.[57]

No mere empiricist, the new professor soon 'excited more public interest than his medical school'.[58] Halford vigorously critiqued Thomas Huxley's 1863 *Evidence as to Man's Place in Nature* for extending Darwin's theory of natural selection to *Homo sapiens*. When the arrival of the first gorillas in Melbourne in 1865 saw Halford branding Huxley 'the devil', he was keelhauled by the British medical press as Darwinian converts multiplied.[59] However sincere his providentialist natural theology, Halford's differentiation between 'man' and gorilla also carried overt ethical implications. Having built his reputation on vivisection, Halford doubtless appreciated his animal subjects as sentient beings. Once he began employing them for snake venom studies, however, 'Professor Halford's dogs' became political, professional and epistemological actors in the fractious medical climate of mid-century Victoria.

Hybrid cells: the germ theory of snake poisoning

A feared but rarely fatal accident, snakebite was blamed for 45 deaths across Victoria over 1864–74.[60] Little wonder that Burstall's dissolution in the colonial capital – especially involving an exotic serpent – occasioned medical and media interest. Amongst those attending the autopsy was Halford, who had previously encountered venomous snakes in India and documented the rare phenomenon of an adder bite in Britain. Given the cobra, he killed it and tested its venom upon a dog, which 'died after the usual symptoms during the same night'.[61]

Having inspected Burstall's 'fluid alkaline dark blood', Halford's microscopic survey of the dog's blood led him to generate an entirely new entity. He was struck by the millions of 'nucleated cells of a perfectly circular form ... [containing a] remarkable spot ... distinctly visible in all'. He found similar cells, albeit lacking the macula, in the venom of the cobra and an Australian black snake, which he tested upon the blood of a sacrificed dog, kitten, pigeon and rat. Taking the exponential multiplication of these microscopic phenomena to imply that they comprised living 'germinal matter' from the snake, Halford postulated that their interaction with host cells might produce 'a hybrid nucleated maculated cell, except for its circular form, like a reptile's blood corpuscle'.[62]

This was a remarkable hypothesis. Halford theorised that the nucleated cells comprised an animal 'virus', a term synonymous with venom since the eighteenth century. It implied furthermore a substance manufactured in the body in response to disease, becoming itself an agent of infection. Indeed, Halford considered it a zymotic process, in the mould of Pasteur's ferments. Pairing his microscopic observations with the victim's loss of heat, plus the dearth of oxygen and clotting agent in the blood, he surmised that 'oxidation of the food in the blood and of the tissues is transferred from the bitten man to the foreign cell, which is equivalent to saying, that *animal power is transferred from the one to the other*'.[63] Envenomation, Halford postulated, spawned a victim–snake hybrid, a fecund population of parasitical cells that swarmed in the bloodstream to drain the victim's 'animal power'. Rendering these entities 'real' by illustrating them for scientific audiences (Figure 15), Halford's ontology appeared to dissolve the species boundaries his anti-Darwinian arguments had attempted to bolster.[64]

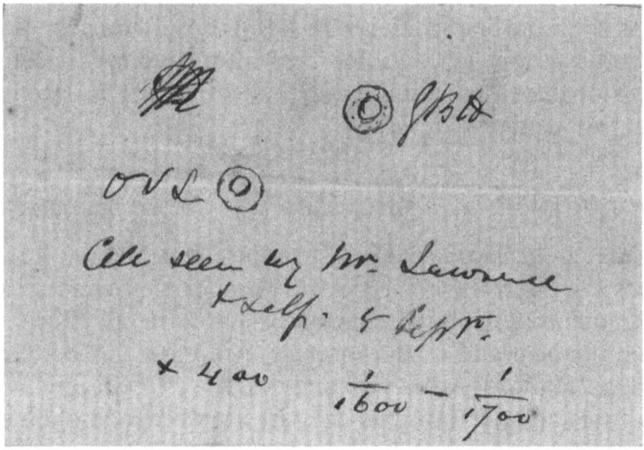

15 George B. Halford, 'Cell seen by Mr. Lawrence & self', 5 September 1867.

Emboldened by his handful of experiments and a scaffold of conjecture, Halford allied his observations to those of famed German pathologist Rudolf Virchow. Musing whether 'this eminent man has mistaken foreign cells for the white corpuscles', he invoked other authors who considered cholera another poison that potently diminished 'animal heat'. 'It cannot be unreasonable to suppose that as both the symptoms and *post-mortem* appearances in severe cases of cholera and snake-poisoning are nearly identical, they may have a *kindred* origin.' Indeed,

> if we consider that the dried poison of the cobra has been kept for ten years and then destroyed life by inoculation, and remember that the home of cholera and of the cobra and other venomous reptiles is India, and that millions of reptiles die yearly, and then as pollen is carried from place to place by insects, so may this dried poison be ... and subsequently inhaled ... therefore no poison-fang is needed [to] kill a man in a little more than five minutes.[65]

In short, Halford proposed, the origin of cholera might be the desiccated venom of innumerable deceased snakes, wafting from the subcontinent to contaminate the atmosphere 'in the same way as the germs of hydatid disease were known to'.[66] Such 'cholera clouds', note both Dhrub Kumar Singh and Projit Mukharji, served as synecdoches for the insidious diffusion of Indian 'poisons' into western bodies and geographies. Furthermore their protean existence as 'objects without an essence' paralleled the historical ontology of Halford's germinal matter, foreshadowing 'the tensions of the emergent global culture: pulled between deterritorialized uniformity and obstinate local specificity, between the lure of the exotic and the fear of the unknown, between the impossibility of the supernatural and the spiritual depletion of the natural'.[67]

Intercolonial circuits of exchange

Thus did a fatal bite by a Ceylonese cobra in Melbourne trigger a protracted circuit of intercolonial exchange. Typical of the transmissive tenor of the times was a letter outlining Halford's 'germinal matter' observations. First appearing in the Melbourne *Argus* on 26 April 1867, it was facsimiled or extracted in countless colonial newspapers, plus the *Transactions and Proceedings of the Royal Society of Victoria*, the *Australian Medical Journal*, London's *Medical Times and Gazette* and the *New York Medical Journal*.[68] Indeed, remarked Philadelphia physiologist Silas Weir Mitchell, 'this strange theory has been copied widely without comment in medical journals ... I have been asked by many physicians if it were correct.'[69] In his estimation, it was not. As Mitchell asserted, the 'masses of germinal matter described by Professor Halford have no actual existence, so far as the rattlesnake is concerned at least'.[70]

Nevertheless, Halford had stirred a global pot. When a variant of his letter appeared in the *British Medical Journal*, it soon excited readers in the Indian Medical Service. 'The subject of cobra poison', recorded Charles Francis, Surgeon Major in the Bengal Army, 'is now attracting a considerable amount of attention in the profession in India and Australia. It is one of the highest importance in a physiological sense, and popularly as terrifying as cholera.'[71] Throughout 1868, rebuttals of Halford's research appeared regularly in the *Indian Medical Gazette*, recombined into a new series for the *Edinburgh Medical Journal*, then selectively twisted for readers of the anti-Halford *Australian Medical Gazette*.[72] By 1869 Mitchell expostulated that 'snakebites and the toxicology of venom poisoning have of late attracted so much attention in English Medical journals' that he felt compelled to chide Indian and Australian interlocutors for not 'examining the subject with all the aids now familiar to the modern toxicologist'.[73]

Halford's germinal matter theory commanded such ubiquity precisely for its presumed universality. Both snakebite and cholera were typified by random distribution, calamitous onset and fatal sequelae. Fear of such urgent, entropic demise haunted Britons during cholera epidemics; likewise, cobras continued to enjoy an Imperial notoriety telegraphed by the London Zoo case of 1852.[74] If venom and cholera were fundamentally linked, Halford queried, 'may we not hope to know something definite of the poisons of hydrophobia, small-pox, scarlet fever, and, indeed, of all zymotic diseases?'[75]

Indeed, from the late 1850s it was increasingly accepted that cholera was attributable to a specific, possibly contagious, agent.[76] In his 1860 monograph, Mitchell himself had drawn attention to 'the singular likeness between the symptoms and lesions of Crotalus [rattlesnake] poisoning, and those of certain maladies, such as yellow fever … cholera, typhoid, and typhus fevers, and in scarlatina'.[77] Thus although cholera never reached nineteenth-century Australia, there was no immediate reason why Halford's theorem should sink into what Christopher Hamlin coins 'the black hole that swallowed cholera publications'.[78]

Keeping germinal matter alive

Locally, Halford's 'striking discovery' inspired only fleeting interest. Throughout 1867, he continued experimenting upon dogs and cats, exhausting his cache of cobra venom. To bolster his status as an expert microscopist, he presented fresh observations to the Royal Society of Victoria, reinforcing the elusive essence of his phenomenon: '*As the cells increase the nebulous germinal matter disappears*'.[79] Injecting venom into a pregnant cat, Halford declared the death of the mother and her foetal kittens doubly significant. Transmission of the poisonous particles across the allantoic membrane demonstrated their 'extreme minuteness', while affirming 'that the path of snake-venom, syphilis, small-pox, and other poisons are much alike, each passes from the mother to the young – each passes from one organism to another'.[80] Conveying these results to the *British Medical Journal*, eminent pathologist James Paget subjoined a proviso: 'the facts are very strange – so strange, that it may be well for me to add that Professor Halford, writing to me, says, that I may "depend on the patience and fear of error" with which he has worked at them'.[81]

Halford hardly lacked influential allies. When the Duke of Edinburgh visited Melbourne University on 3 January 1868, its medical professor impressed him with a dead dog. His Royal Highness proved less attentive, however, to Halford's explanation that it had been killed by germinal matter injected by a snake.[82] Delivering his 1868 Anniversary Address as President of the Royal Society of Victoria, Government Astronomer Robert Ellery affirmed that 'those who have carefully observed the blood in snake-poisoned individuals, cannot … be in the least doubt as to the fact of the presence of these cells. My friend and I were very sceptical on this point, and at first failed to see them.'[83] The friend was George Foord, assayer for Melbourne's Royal Mint. 'Two of the most scientific men in Melbourne', Halford asserted, who yet wasted an afternoon seeking germinal matter in the blood of a snakebitten dog until he arrived and 'at once saw hundreds of the cells as well formed as could be'. Soon his esteemed companions 'saw just as many as I could see myself'.[84]

While such potent corroboration bolstered the ontological status of germinal matter, Halford's correlation between snake poison and cholera found few Victorian converts. Thomas Ralph, surgeon and soon-to-be founder of the colony's Microscopical Society, argued that Prussic acid produced similar effects on blood. James Neild, President of the Medical Society of Victoria and Editor of the *Australian Medical Journal*, concurred that Halford had not provided 'sufficient proof of the germ increasing'.[85]

Yet his germinal matter flourished across the Australian colonies.[86] Geelong surgeon John Day opined in September 1868 that the professor's theory might also apply to the poison of diphtheria.[87] Halford's most fervent proselyte was (George) Hogarth Pringle, a Parramatta surgeon who rightly claimed to have been the first in Australia to apply Joseph Lister's antiseptic principles to wound management.[88] Formerly serving at the Edinburgh Cholera Hospital and with the British Army in the Crimea, Pringle was acquainted with cholera 'in all its stages'.[89] Having also witnessed snakebites in America, India, Ceylon and New South Wales, he asserted that the 'causes of death … in cholera and snake-bite are identical, and this theory of molecular or cellular growth is the only one that will fairly account for the *post-mortem* movements observed in the former disease'.[90] Into 1871, Victorian surgeon John Stuart forwarded a blood sample from a snakebite victim. His hand-drawn sketches of the 'maculate corpuscles', however, represented the last local observations keeping Halford's microscopic germinal matter 'alive'.[91]

A gift squandered: the transnational demise of germinal matter

While Halford increasingly courted such parochial supporters, he equally anticipated 'much good resulting from East Indians, Americans, and Australians working contemporaneously at the subjects before us'.[92] Indeed, the resultant transcolonial exchanges – and their escalation into the 1870s as detailed in the next chapter – profoundly question Chakrabarti's claim that nineteenth-century venom research in British India 'reflected the characteristics of colonial science defined by the metropolis and the periphery'.[93]

Materialising the potency of 'peripheral' networks, in February 1868 Mitchell wrote to Halford, reiterating that his careful examinations had identified no germinal matter in the envenomed blood of various creatures. Accompanying this missive was a pill-box containing dried rattlesnake venom. 'Desirous to offer you a chance of fairly comparing results', he proposed, 'Can you not send me specimens in like manner of the dry venom of your own serpents?'[94]

The offer was never reciprocated. Halford, however, eagerly exploited his windfall: 'examining the dried poison of the *rattlesnake*, previously dissolved in warm water, the microscopic appearances noted by me were – minute spherical particles of germinal matter, and ... larger free nuclei'.[95] Curiously, although Mitchell had earlier contemplated that rattlesnake venom might be a 'septic or putrefacient poison of astounding energy', Halford did not connect these proposals to his own zymotic theories of venom activity.[96]

If Halford's recalcitrance sabotaged this potential ontological concordance, his results inspired Mitchell to question its variability. Hitherto, he had presumed that since the venoms of the viper, rattlesnake and American copperhead displayed identical toxic activities, Indian cobra poison would act similarly. However, following Halford's claim that envenomation by the Australian tiger snake produced no local symptoms at the bite site – unlike cobra or rattlesnake bites – Mitchell besought 'other observers in British India and Australia' to 'enable us to know if the venom of various serpents be identical in form and force of toxic action or not'.[97]

Officers of the Indian Medical Service were not remiss. Seeking an antidote to cobra venom, John Shortt – Superintendent-General of Vaccine in the Madras Presidency – posted a reward which by 1868 had reached a princely £175.[98] His studies of cobra venom in dogs, horses and quails led Shortt to admit, with a nod to Halford, that 'poisoned blood shows under the microscope a peculiar notched appearance, and apparently what appeared to be small granules. It requires further research with a more powerful microscope than I can at present command.'[99]

The quantity and quality of microscopical observations suffused Joseph Fayrer's exhaustive studies of Indian snake venoms. As Professor of Surgery at the Medical College of Bengal, over 1867–71 he explored cobra, king cobra, daboia and banded krait venoms, inoculating them back into these venomous serpents, plus the innocuous rat snake, yellow monitor lizard, snails, frogs, fish, pigeons, fowls, pigs, horses, domestic canines and semi-wild 'pariah dogs'.[100] Compared with Halford's sporadic, anecdotal and largely solitary observations, Fayrer constantly reiterated the technical capacities of his microscopes and the expertise of his corroborating colonial observers.

This fastidiousness is curious: Fayrer later noted that his interest in snake venoms coincided with a growing scepticism over bacillary theories of disease.[101] Yet in 1868, he professed being 'in favour of the theory advocated' by Halford.[102] Fayrer made no comment on the putative cholera link, but faithfully reported several instances in which cobra poisoning generated apparent germinal matter in blood samples.[103] Such observations were never uniform, however, being outweighed by the plethora of contrary results. At best, he accorded 'germinal matter' a partial role in explaining protracted deaths following snakebite. Like his American counterpart, Mitchell, Fayrer could not apprehend how the purported multiplication of millions of invasive, hybridising cells could explain deaths among envenomed animals in under two minutes.[104]

Halford's antipodean antagonists crowed that 'no observer, either in Europe or elsewhere, has been able to verify Professor Halford's so-called discovery anent the alleged alteration of the corpuscles of the blood in cases of snake-poisoning'.[105] Yet until 1873, he remained the only investigator worldwide able to experiment with the venoms of the Indian cobra, the American rattlesnake and Australian ophidians. As early as October 1868 he ventured a double gambit:

> We have arrived at a point where a difference seems to exist between the effects of the poison of the *tiger snake* and that of both the *cobra* and the *rattlesnake* ... the venom fangs ... in the *cobra* and *rattlesnake* are strong and large, those in the *tiger snake* small. From this, and from experiment, I infer that the poison of the latter is as deadly as, or even more so than, that of the former snake. In the cases of death by either, the microscopic and physical conditions of the blood are similar.[106]

Quite simply, Halford proposed that Australian snakes possessed venom more virulent than the world's two most feared serpents. Nevertheless, by 1868 his putative linkage between venom and the 'germs' of cholera was effectively moribund. Both Charles Campbell and Sharon Wallace suggest that – however poorly received – Halford's attempts to incorporate emerging strands of germ theory into antipodean medical epistemology were laudable.[107] It was a more generous assessment than Geoffrey Blainey's lament that Halford's investigative expertise of was 'a gift squandered in futile research'.[108]

The productive power of ontological agents

However vainglorious his intent, the transcolonial networks Halford mobilised in 1867–68 were incredibly productive. They circulated, refracted and connected 'germinal matter' to observers in Britain, Bengal, Philadelphia and the Australian hinterland, briefly generating a new ontological possibility. Perhaps the venom of snakes, and by extension the poison of many dread diseases, comprised an evanescent yet potent animal substance that colonised, hybridised and ultimately exhausted the 'animal power' of its host. Although soon derided, Halford's conceptualisation of this 'virus' was surprisingly similar to the nosology of filterable viral diseases that emerged in the 1920s.[109]

This is not to suggest that he was ahead of his time. Halford's desire to locate obligate parasites within snake venom paralleled his contemporaries' erratic investment in similar ontological agents of disease.[110] Nevertheless, amidst the 'germs' and then 'bacteria' that proliferated from 1865 to 1900, the productive power that Halford imputed to 'germinal matter' was beguiling. 'It abounds in the secretions from the glands, in the head of the spermatozoon, in salavine and pepsine, in the chyle-corpuscle, white corpuscle, pus globule, tubercle, syphitis, cancers pre-eminently, vaccine, small-pox, mildew, and in microscopic parasites of all kinds, &c.', he enthused. 'Marvellous are the results brought about by its presence.'[111]

But testimony alone was insufficient: Latour insists that Pasteur was never just 'the revealer of microbes'.[112] As the failed case of rabies in Hobart Town affirmed, clinical conviction and localised authority counted for little. For a novel animal poison – or indeed any aetiological agent – to garner ontological credence, actors had to be multiplied, networks mobilised and performances convincingly repeated. Only thus could snake germs be *made* real.

What Halford saw was occasionally witnessed by others in Australia and India, if not America. Yet 'germinal matter' formed just one component of the assemblage. Equally important was apparatus: the microscopes which represented the common material element linking disparate scientific sites. But, as Ian Hacking argues, practitioners 'learn to see through a microscope by doing, not just by looking'.[113] Localised craft knowledges determined whether or not international investigators could 'see' Halford's putatively universal phenomenon.[114]

Yet the fact that so many repeatedly sought to replicate his findings only confirms that, ontologically, germinal matter 'existed' – at least until 1871. Just as Victoria's Government Astronomer confessed to at first 'failing' to see germinal cells, Fayrer himself admitted in 1868 that 'up to the present time, I have been *unable to discover* the blood changes described by Professor Halford'.[115] His remark betrays a professional courtesy, certainly, but also an ontological possibilism.

Unlike Hobart Town's rabid spaniel, animal participants were rarely foregrounded in the germinal matter controversy. If microscopy could not confirm that venoms were 'alive', Halford's vivisections granted them a unique character. Like snakes, venoms now comprised discrete species, characterised by pathognomonic toxicities and geographical particularities.[116] But to prove this assertion, investigators paradoxically had to assert that their animal victims were interchangeable – that a Philadelphia stray facsimiled a Bombay 'pariah dog'.

Translocating apparatus, however, did not necessarily stabilise what investigators *saw*. Mitchell himself confessed in 1869 that neither venoms nor victims were uniform: 'I know of no other poison the activity of which seems to be more distinctly affected by the individual peculiarities of the animal poisoned'.[117] The ongoing unease over rabies, and exactly which dogs might prove susceptible to its elusive agent, reinforced this uncertainty. For all of the attempts of scientific medicine to stress their fungibility, animals remained sentient individuals.

The consequences were both existential and moral. Ultimately, the boundary most threatened by Halford's germinal matter was not colonial, nor even Imperial. What was truly alarming was the prospect of transubstantiation: the conversion of human tissue into an interspecies hybrid dominated by its primitive, reptilian character. As early as the 1660s it was theorised that blood transfusion between species – including humans – might alter the humoral constitution of the recipient.[118] The possibility that animal contamination might comprise microscopic bodies was neither novel nor innocuous, as contemporaneous antivaccinationist agitation attested.[119]

Within the colonial animal matrix, dangerous creatures disturbed Victorian sensibilities not just because they resisted human dominance. As with the enduring moral opprobrium inhering in bestiality, they represented a declensionist fear of consubstantiality, the melding of human and animal.[120] Thomas Bowring was heard to bark like a dog as he succumbed to hydrophobia; when bitten by his cobra, John Burstall's keening likewise resembled the whine of a hound. A similar fear of slippage between civilised and 'savage' characterised mid-Victorian fears of cholera.[121] Despite his vigorous dismissal of Darwinism, the germinal matter purveyed by Halford posed an analogous ontological threat. Rather than evolutionary progress, however, this rapacious reptilian poison represented a fearful portent of atavism in an era of growing human identification with the 'brute creation'.

Notes

1 Owsei Temkin, 'The scientific approach to disease: specific entity and individual sickness', in A.C. Crombie (ed.), *Scientific Change: Historical Studies in the Intellectual, Social, and Technical Conditions for Scientific Discovery and Technical Invention, from Antiquity to the Present* (London: Heinemann, 1963), pp. 629–47.

2 David N. Livingstone, *Putting Science in its Place: Geographies of Scientific Knowledge* (Chicago: University of Chicago Press, 2003), pp. 12, 185.

3 Thomas S. Kuhn, *The Structure of Scientific Revolutions*, 2nd edn (Chicago: University of Chicago Press, 1970), p. 26.
4 Ian Hacking, *Historical Ontology* (Cambridge, Mass.: Harvard University Press, 2002), p. 23.
5 Tony Bennett, *Anthropological Assemblages: Producing Culture as a Surface of Government* (Milton Keynes: Centre for Research on Socio-Cultural Change, 2008), pp. 2–5.
6 Lorraine Daston, 'On scientific observation', *Isis*, 99:1 (2008), pp. 98, 107.
7 'Dissertation on the snake wound – continued', *Sydney Gazette and New South Wales Advertiser* (13 November 1819), p. 4; William Boag, 'On the poison of serpents', *Asiatick Researches*, 6 (1801), pp. 120–6.
8 William Bland, 'To the Editor of the *Sydney Gazette*', *Sydney Gazette and New South Wales Advertiser* (28 October 1826), p. 4.
9 L.E.L., 'To the Editor of the *Sydney Gazette*', *Sydney Gazette and New South Wales Advertiser* (4 November 1826), p. 4.
10 H. Schlegel, *Essay on the Physiognomy of Serpents*, trans. Thos. Stewart Traill (Edinburgh: Stewart and Co., 1843), p. 49.
11 James Apjohn, 'Toxicology', in John Forbes, Alexander Tweedie, and John Conolly (eds), *The Cyclopædia of Practical Medicine*, vol. 4 (London: Sherwood, Gilbert, and Piper, and Baldwin and Cradock, 1835), pp. 189, 222.
12 Clement Hodgkinson, 'Poison of snakes', *Age* (15 December 1868), p. 3.
13 *Ibid.*
14 Clement Hodgkinson, *Australia, from Port Macquarie to Moreton Bay; with Descriptions of the Natives, Their Manners and Customs; the Geology, Natural Productions, Fertility, and Resources of That Region* (London: T. and W. Boone, 1845), pp. 212–13.
15 Robert Lehane, *Duelling Surgeon, Colonial Patriot: The Remarkable Life of William Bland* (North Melbourne: Australian Scholarly Publishing, 2011), pp. 69–70; W. Bland, 'Report of a case of snake-bite, with observations on the treatment in such instances', *Lancet*, 51:1272 (1848), p. 72.
16 James W. Agnew, 'Notes on the teeth and poison apparatus of the snakes of Tasman's Peninsula', *Tasmanian Journal of Natural Science, Agriculture, Statistics, &c.*, 2:8 (1846), pp. 197, 199–200.
17 Alfred Roberts, 'On the structure and functions of the venom apparatus in serpents', *Sydney Magazine of Science and Art*, 1 (1858), p. 130.
18 Alfred Roberts, 'On the structure and function of the poison apparatus in venomous serpents, with a description of some of the species found in Australia', *Sydney Magazine of Science and Art*, 2 (1859), p. 53.
19 Harriet Ritvo, *The Animal Estate: The English and Other Creatures in the Victorian Age* (Cambridge, Mass.: Harvard University Press, 1987), p. 13.
20 See Harriet Ritvo, 'Zoological nomenclature and the empire of Victorian science', in Bernard Lightman (ed.), *Victorian Science in Context* (Chicago: University of Chicago Press, 1997), pp. 334–53; Mario A. Di Gregorio, 'In search of the natural system: problems of zoological classification in Victorian Britain', *History and Philosophy of the Life Sciences*, 4 (1982), pp. 227–54.
21 Roberts, 'On the structure and function of the poison apparatus in venomous serpents', p. 53.
22 Michael Worboys, *Spreading Germs: Disease Theories and Medical Practice in Britain, 1865–1900* (Cambridge: Cambridge University Press, 2000), pp. 32–6.
23 C. Ball, 'Joseph Clover and the cobra: a tale of snake envenomation and attempted resuscitation with bellows in London, 1852', *Anaesthesia and Intensive Care*, 38:1 (2010), pp. 5–9.
24 Albert E. Gunther, *A Century of Zoology at the British Museum through the Lives of Two Keepers, 1815–1914* (London: Dawsons, 1975), pp. 299–301.
25 Pratik Chakrabarti, *Bacteriology in British India: Laboratory Medicine and the Tropics* (Rochester: University of Rochester Press, 2012), p. 116.
26 Kay Anderson, 'Culture and nature at the Adelaide Zoo: at the frontiers of

"human" geography', *Transactions of the Institute of British Geographers*, 20:3 (1995), p. 281.

27 John Simons, *The Tiger That Swallowed the Boy: Exotic Animals in Victorian England* (Oxfordshire: Libri Publishing, 2012), pp. 39–40.

28 See Albert Günther, 'Fourth account of new species of snakes in the collection of the British Museum', *Annals and Magazine of Natural History*, 15 (third series):86 (1865), pp. 89–98.

29 E. Swarbreck Hall, 'On snake bites', *Australian Medical Journal*, 4 (1859), p. 96.

30 Elsie Frances Haynes, 'Edward Swarbreck Hall: medical scientist and social reformer in colonial Tasmania' (MA thesis, University of Tasmania, 1976), pp. 224–5.

31 Roberts, 'On the structure and function of the poison apparatus in venomous serpents', p. 53.

32 J.W. Agnew, 'Notes on the poison of venomous snakes', *Papers and Proceedings of the Royal Society of Tasmania* (1864), p. 9.

33 See Margaret Pelling, 'The meaning of contagion: reproduction, medicine and metaphor', in Alison Bashford and Claire Hooker (eds), *Contagion: Epidemics, History and Culture from Smallpox to Anthrax* (Annandale: Pluto Press, 2002), p. 22.

34 Daniel Sennert, Nicholas Culpeper and Abdiah Cole, *The Sixth Book of Practical Physick of Occult or Hidden Diseases* (London: Peter Cole, 1662), p. 14. See also George M. Baer, 'The history of rabies', in Alan C. Jackson and William H. Wunner (eds), *Rabies*, 2nd edn (Amsterdam: Elsevier, 2007), pp. 1–7.

35 Ritvo, *The Animal Estate*, pp. 168–73, 184.

36 James Boyce, *Van Diemen's Land* (Melbourne: Black, 2008), p. 183.

37 Neil Pemberton and Michael Worboys, *Mad Dogs and Englishmen: Rabies in Britain, 1830–2000* (Houndmills: Palgrave Macmillan, 2007), p. 76.

38 Thos. C. Smart and E. Swarbreck Hall, 'Hydrophobia in Hobart Town', *Australian Medical Journal*, 12 (1867), pp. 166–7, 176.

39 *Ibid.*, pp. 168, 172.

40 *Ibid.*, p. 172.

41 Rebecca Kippen, 'Rabies in Tasmania', *Chainletter*, 3 (December 2009), pp. 4–5; W.E.L.H. Crowther, 'A case of so-called hydrophobia: a matter of diagnosis', *Medical Journal of Australia*, 1 (1946), pp. 69–72; Ian Parsonson, *The Australian Ark: A History of Domesticated Animals in Australia* (Collingwood: CSIRO Publishing, 2000), pp. 238–9.

42 Smart and Hall, 'Hydrophobia in Hobart Town', pp. 181–2.

43 Crowther, 'A case of so-called hydrophobia', p. 72.

44 John Hunter, 'Observations, and heads of inquiry, on canine madness, drawn from the cases and materials collected by the Society, respecting that disease', *Transactions of a Society for the Improvement of Medical and Chirurgical Knowledge*, I (1793), pp. 324–5; Lise Wilkinson, 'John Hunter and the transmissibility of rabies', *Veterinary History*, 2 (new series 2) (1981–82), pp. 79–81.

45 Karen Brown, *Mad Dogs and Meerkats: A History of Resurgent Rabies in Southern Africa* (Cape Town: University of Cape Town Press, 2011), pp. 20–37.

46 Harriet Ritvo, 'Animals in nineteenth-century Britain: complicated attitudes and competing categories', in Aubrey Manning and James Serpell (eds), *Animals and Human Society: Changing Perspectives* (London: Routledge, 1994), p. 110.

47 P.J. Macwhirter, 'Shifting paradigms: the hard road to acceptance of the contagion principle in Australia', *Australian Veterinary Journal*, 75:7 (1997), pp. 517–18.

48 Eric Rolls, *A Million Wild Acres: 200 Years of Man and an Australian Forest* (Melbourne: Thomas Nelson Australia, 1981), pp. 169, 174.

49 Bruno Latour, *The Pasteurization of France*, trans. Alan Sheridan and John Law (Cambridge, Mass.: Harvard University Press, 1988), p. 83.

50 Bruno Latour, *On the Modern Cult of the Factish Gods*, trans. Catherine Porter and Heather MacLean (Durham: Duke University Press, 2010), pp. 19–20.

51 Bruno Latour, 'On the partial existence of existing and nonexisting objects', in

Lorraine Daston (ed.), *Biographies of Scientific Objects* (Chicago: University of Chicago Press, 2000), p. 257.

52 See Iwan Rhys Morus, 'Worlds of wonder: sensation and the Victorian scientific performance', *Isis*, 101:4 (2010), pp. 806–16.

53 'The fatal snake accident', *Queanbeyan Age and General Advertiser* (26 April 1867), p. 2.

54 'Death from the bite of a cobra-di-capella', *Argus* (15 April 1867), p. 5.

55 University of Melbourne Archives, Melbourne (hereafter UMA), 1981.0062, Halford, George Britton, 'Letters to Professor G. Halford referring to his antidote – injection with ammonia', 1867–1937, Francis Smith Fielder to GB Halford, 24 April 1867, p. 2.

56 W.A. Osborne, 'George Britton Halford: his life and work', *Medical Journal of Australia*, 1 (1929), p. 65.

57 G.B. Halford, 'University of Melbourne. Medical School', *Medical & Surgical Review (Australasian)*, I (1863), pp. 88–9; J.E. Neild, 'The Medical School of the University of Melbourne', *Speculum* 46 (1900), pp. 3–4.

58 Geoffrey Blainey, *A Centenary History of the University of Melbourne* (Melbourne: Melbourne University Press, 1957), p. 28.

59 Barry W. Butcher, 'Gorilla warfare in Melbourne: Halford, Huxley and "Man's place in nature"', in R.W. Home (ed.), *Australian Science in the Making* (Cambridge: Cambridge University Press, 1988), pp. 164–7; Ross L. Jones, *Humanity's Mirror: 150 Years of Anatomy in Melbourne* (South Yarra: Haddington Press, 2007), p. 39.

60 Victorian Humane Society, *First Annual Report* (Melbourne: Victorian Humane Society, 1875), p. 6.

61 George B. Halford, 'On the condition of the blood after death from snake-bite, as a probable clue to the further study of zymotic diseases, and of cholera especially', *Transactions and Proceedings of the Royal Society of Victoria*, 8 (1868), p. 75.

62 *Ibid.*, pp. 76, 78.

63 *Ibid.*, p. 85. Italics in original.

64 See Harriet Ritvo, 'Border trouble: shifting the line between people and other animals', *Social Research*, 62:3 (1995), pp. 491–5.

65 Halford, 'On the condition of the blood after death from snake-bite', pp. 91–2. Italics in original.

66 'Local topics', *Australian Medical Journal*, 12 (1867), p. 221.

67 Projit Bihari Mukharji, 'The "cholera cloud" in the nineteenth-century "British world": history of an object-without-an-essence', *Bulletin of the History of Medicine*, 86:3 (2012), p. 332; see also Dhrub Kumar Singh, '"Clouds of cholera" and clouds around cholera, 1817–70', in Deepak Kumar (ed.), *Disease and Medicine in India: A Historical Overview* (Aligarh: Indian History Congress, 2001), pp. 144–65.

68 George B. Halford, 'Experiments on the poison of the cobra-di-capella', *Argus* (26 April 1867), p. 6.

69 S.W. Mitchell, 'Experimental contributions to the toxicology of rattle-snake venom', *New York Medical Journal*, 6:4 (1868), pp. 311–12.

70 'Snake poison', *Medical Times and Gazette*, 2 (new series 37) (1868), p. 249.

71 Charles R. Francis, 'On the action of cobra poison', *Indian Medical Gazette*, 3 (1868), p. 73.

72 To cite merely one example, J. Fayrer, 'On the action of the cobra poison – second series', *Indian Medical Gazette*, 3 (1868), pp. 74–5, formed the basis for J. Fayrer, 'On the action of the cobra poison (continued)', *Edinburgh Medical Journal*, 14 (part II) (1869), pp. 915–23, which was in turn reconfigured as Dr Fayrer, 'The action of the cobra poison', *Australian Medical Gazette*, 1 (1869), pp. 132–4.

73 S. Weir Mitchell, 'The venom of serpents', *Medical Times and Gazette*, 38 (1869), p. 138.

74 W.J. Moore, 'A case of snake-bite', *Indian Medical Gazette*, 3 (1868), p. 104; Margaret Pelling, *Cholera, Fever and English Medicine* (Oxford: Oxford University Press, 1978), pp. 4–5.

75 George B. Halford, 'Experiments on the poison of the cobra-di-capella', *British Medical Journal*, 2:342 (1867), p. 44.
76 Singh, '"Clouds of cholera" and clouds around cholera', pp. 150–2.
77 S. Weir Mitchell, *Researches Upon the Venom of the Rattlesnake: With an Investigation of the Anatomy and Physiology of the Organs Concerned* (Philadelphia: Collins, 1860), p. 97.
78 Christopher Hamlin, *Cholera: The Biography* (Oxford: Oxford University Press, 2009), p. 191.
79 G.B. Halford, 'White corpuscles of blood or germ cells', *Australasian* (22 February 1868), p. 251. Italics in original.
80 *Ibid.*
81 G.B. Halford, 'Further observations on the condition of the blood after death from snake-bite', *British Medical Journal*, 2:364 (1867), p. 563.
82 Blainey, *A Centenary History of the University of Melbourne*, p. 36.
83 R.L.J. Ellery, 'Anniversary address of the President', *Transactions and Proceedings of the Royal Society of Victoria*, 9 (1868), pp. 7–8.
84 George B. Halford, 'Snake-poisoning and its treatment (continued)', *Medical Times and Gazette*, 2 (new series 47) (1873), p. 171.
85 Thomas Shearman Ralph, 'Observations on the action of snake poison on the blood', *Australian Medical Journal*, 12 (1867), p. 361.
86 See Sharon Louise Wallace, 'Treatment of snakebite from Halford to Sutherland' (BMedSci thesis, University of Melbourne, 1983), pp. 41, 118–19.
87 John Day, 'On diphtheria', *Australian Medical Journal*, 13 (1868), p. 269.
88 Iain Macintyre, 'George (1830–72) and his son James Hogarth (1863–1941) Pringle: unsung surgical pioneers', *Journal of Medical Biography*, 16:3 (2008), p. 156.
89 UMA 1981.0062, G Hogarth Pringle to GB Halford, 30 April 1867, p. 3.
90 G. Hogarth Pringle, 'The blood in snake-poisoning', *Australian Medical Journal*, 13 (1868), p. 286.
91 UMA, Melbourne, 1981.0062, Halford, George Britton, 'Newspaper cuttings relating to snake-bite and antidote i.e. ammonia (Prof G.B. Halford)', 1867–1876, John Stuart to GB Halford, 11 January 1871 [incorrectly dated 1870] and 12 January 1871.
92 George B. Halford, 'On snake-poisoning', *Australasian* ([October?] 1868), n.p.
93 Chakrabarti, *Bacteriology in British India*, p. 124.
94 UMA 1981.0062, Silas Weir Mitchell to GB Halford, 28 February 1868.
95 Halford, 'On snake-poisoning', n.p. Italics in original.
96 Mitchell, *Researches Upon the Venom of the Rattlesnake*, p. 95.
97 Mitchell, 'The venom of serpents', p. 137.
98 Francis, 'On the action of cobra poison', p. 73.
99 John Shortt, 'Experiments with the poison of the cobra di capella', *Lancet*, 91:2333 (1868), pp. 616–17.
100 See Barbara J. Hawgood, 'Sir Joseph Fayrer MD FRS (1824–1907) Indian Medical Service: snakebite and mortality in British India', *Toxicon*, 34:2 (1996), pp. 174–5.
101 Joseph Fayrer, *Recollections of My Life* (Edinburgh: William Blackwood and Sons, 1900), p. 281.
102 J. Fayrer, 'Experiments on the influence of snake-poison (continued)', *Indian Medical Gazette*, 3 (1868), p. 265.
103 For instance, J. Fayrer, 'On the action of the cobra venom', *Edinburgh Medical Journal*, 14 (part I) (1868), p. 525.
104 J. Fayrer, 'Experiments on the influence of snake-poison (continued)', p. 265.
105 'Professor Halford and the treatment of snake-poison', *Australian Medical Gazette*, I (1869), p. 265.
106 Halford, 'On snake-poisoning', n.p. Italics in original.
107 C.H. Campbell, 'Professor Halford's germ theory of snake poisoning', *Medical Journal of Australia*, 1 (1966), p. 555; Wallace, 'Treatment of snakebite from Halford to Sutherland', p. 14.

108 Blainey, *A Centenary History of the University of Melbourne*, p. 34.
109 See, for instance, Michael Bresalier, 'Neutralizing flu: "immunological devices" and the making of a virus disease', in Kenton Kroker, Jennifer Keelan and Pauline M.H. Mazumdar (eds), *Crafting Immunity: Working Histories of Clinical Immunology* (Aldershot: Ashgate, 2008), pp. 108–44.
110 Worboys, *Spreading Germs*, pp. 278–81.
111 Halford, 'White corpuscles of blood or germ cells', p. 251.
112 Latour, *The Pasteurization of France*, p. 33.
113 Ian Hacking, 'Do we see through a microscope?', *Pacific Philosophical Quarterly*, 62 (1981), p. 308.
114 See Peter Heering, 'An experimenter's gotta do what an experimenter's gotta do – but how?', *Isis*, 101:4 (2010), pp. 794–805.
115 Fayrer, 'Experiments on the influence of snake-poison (continued)', p. 265. Emphasis mine.
116 See John S. Wilkins, *Species: A History of the Idea* (Berkeley: University of California Press, 2009), pp. 165–80.
117 Mitchell, 'The venom of serpents', p. 137.
118 Douglas Starr, *Blood: An Epic History of Medicine and Commerce* (London: Warner Books, 1999), pp. 11–17.
119 Henry Harris, *The Birth of the Cell* (New Haven: Yale University Press, 2000), pp. 54–9.
120 See for example James Hatley, 'The uncanny goodness of being edible to bears', in Bruce V. Foltz and Robert Frodeman (eds), *Rethinking Nature: Essays in Environmental Philosophy* (Bloomington: Indiana University Press, 2004), p. 21 and Hani Miletski, 'A history of bestiality', in Andrea M. Beetz and Anthony L. Podberscek (eds), *Bestiality and Zoophilia: Sexual Relations with Animals* (Lafayette: Purdue University Press, 2005), pp. 5–9.
121 Erin O'Connor, *Raw Material: Producing Pathology in Victorian Culture* (Durham: Duke University Press, 2000), pp. 34–7, 43–5.

CHAPTER FOUR

In vivo veritas: the amoral ascent of colonial vivisection, 1868–76

'It is pretty well established', asserted the *Hamilton Spectator* on 21 December 1870, 'that a sovereign antidote for the *virus* of the snake has yet to be discovered'. This rural Victorian newspaper nevertheless echoed a common sentiment:

> The subject is one of sufficient importance in a colony like this, to warrant something being done by the State ... A Government Anguinologist (to coin a word), ought to be at least as useful as a Government Palaeontologist, and he might profitably employ his time in trying experiments with the poison of the snake on the lower animals, and also in collecting experiences of its effect on the *genus homo*, when such cases unfortunately arose.[1]

If no official 'Anguinologist' was ever appointed, by 1876 several governments in Australia and India had subsidised snakebite experiments. But more was always at stake than merely effective treatment. Such studies posed a dyadic quandary: was there a cure, and how could it be proven?

This chapter argues that over 1868–76, snakebite experiments transformed more than just colonial understandings of venom. Under contention was the nature of proof, pitting the testimonies of medical gentlemen against envenomed dogs. Polarising the antipodes and the subcontinent, the debate divided professionals and laity, naturalists and doctors, clinicians and experimentalists, rural and urban practitioners. What united them was the hypodermic syringe, a newly popularised technology employed both to study and to treat snakebite. Indeed, by 1876 the process of envenomation was divorced from the event of snakebite, as living creatures themselves became increasingly instrumentalised by medical science.

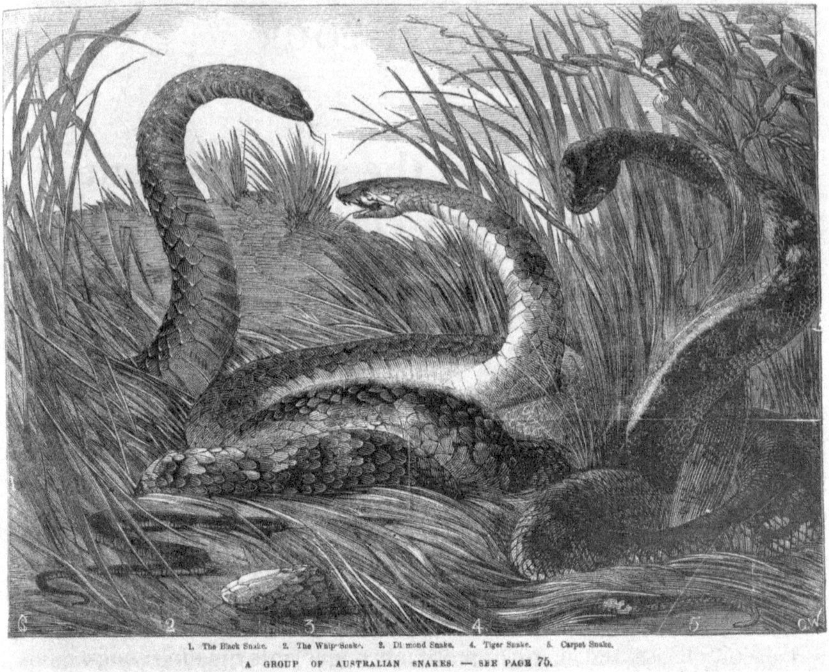

16 Samuel Calvert, 'A group of Australian snakes', *Illustrated Melbourne Post*, 22 May 1868.

Sizing up the snake problem

While snakebite was a receding concern across much of Australia throughout the 1860s, alarm escalated in Victoria, even though its Government Statist calculated a mean annual rate of just 1 snakebite death per 175,000 colonists (Figure 16).[2] An 1876 report indicated that Victorian doctors typically treated 3–4 snakebites over their career, with case-mortality under 10%.[3]

These antipodean disparities paled against Indian epidemiology. A circular seeking reports from hospitals and police stations throughout India and Burma suggested 11,416 snakebite deaths in 1869 alone. Furthermore, opined Joseph Fayrer in collating these data, 'were such information available and collected from the whole of Hindostan, it would be found that more than 20,000 persons die annually from snake-bite' – approximately 1 per 6000 Indian residents.[4] As Pratik Chakrabarti writes, mortality travelled both ways: before 1890, 'most colonial officials believed that destruction of snakes was the only effective and feasible measure to combat the problem'.[5]

Yet with Indian medical journals awash with snakebite reports, Raj fascination with serpents prefigured the investigative culture of tropical medicine.[6] Published over 1796–1809, the authoritative work was Patrick Russell's *An Account of Indian Serpents*, establishing the venomous species 'by the direct method of introducing a live animal into the container and the close observation of clinical signs and symptoms of poisoning'.[7] This work was superseded in 1864 by *The Reptiles of British India*, published by British Museum curator Albert Günther, a physician who asserted that the danger posed by snakebite was largely independent of species.[8]

Günther's monograph inspired Gerard Krefft's *The Snakes of Australia*, self-published in 1869. Director of Sydney's Australian Museum, Krefft frequently experimented upon indigenous frogs, lizards and echidnas, plus cats, dogs and goats (Figure 17).[9] Although unusually attentive to Aboriginal testimony, his hierarchy of danger was dictated by these vivisections. The tiger snake, he decreed, 'is

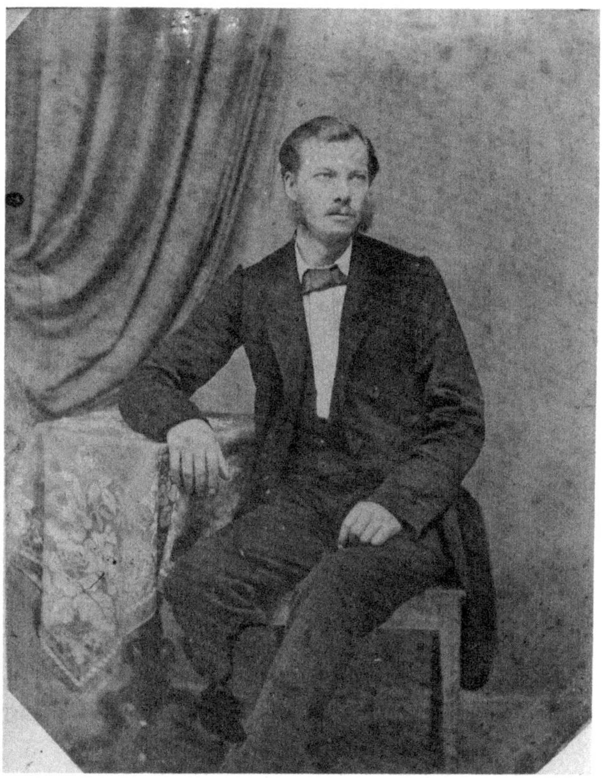

17 Gerard Krefft, *c.*1857.

the most dangerous of all our reptiles, and a fair bite from it will kill animals to the size of a goat in about an a hour'.[10] Nevertheless, as a naturalist, Krefft considered such studies less practical than detailing the distinguishing characteristics of deadly snakes; clinicians seldom demurred.

Colonial practitioners in the public arena

Yet colonial doctors remained a polyglot lot. Typifying their Babel was 'science', a term deployed by literate elites to bolster or challenge governance across the empire, from Melbourne to Malaya.[11] If 'science' held dubious merit for American doctors, in Britain its diverse interpretations denoted membership of specific medical polities.[12] While it proved critical to elevating community perceptions of Victorian doctors by 1900, when George Halford assumed his professorship at Melbourne University in 1863, few words were more divisive in antipodean medical parlance.[13] Indeed, 'scientific medicine' played a promiscuous role in justifying medical fashions and personal idiosyncrasies, often amounting to post-hoc theorisation of treatments for conditions spanning syphilis to snakebite.[14]

If Halford was a prime exponent of this approach, his authority was challenged in 1868 by an arriviste from New South Wales. Boasting a ten-year practice and over a hundred successful cases, ophthalmologist Julius Berncastle asserted that snakebite treatment was so simple that 'a child could do it'.[15] While the crux of his remedy involved removing or cauterising the bitten area, Berncastle's real antidote was at least a pint (570 ml) of spirits – especially brandy – to stimulate flagging patients. Since 1862, he had touted a packet containing a knife, forceps, ligature, lint, sticking-plaster and printed directions. Costing a guinea – nearly a week's average wage – the tin also held a half-pint bottle of his deliberately unpalatable mixture of ammonia and spirits of wine.

In the 1860s, many Imperial doctors, particularly in India, concurred that 'scarifications, suction of the wound, if possible a tight ligature, combined with every means to combat torpor, ought to form the bases of treatment' for snakebite.[16] As the most frequent symptoms after Australian snakebites were vomiting, sleepiness and lassitude, attempts to rouse the patient included frogmarching, firing pistols, shouting, vigorous rubbing, shaking, dousing with cold water, galvanic shocks or merciless flagellation. Beyond occasional amputations, physical measures were similarly haphazard: ligatures, bandaging, cautery, burning or blasting with gunpowder, scarification, suction or leeching. Lay and medical treatments accumulated as the patient's status fluctuated for the first 24 to 48 hours. Ligature was almost universal, although incision or excision of the site remained common. Medicinally, the 'usual remedy' comprised a glass of brandy containing ten drops of strong ammonia – a stimulant and snakebite remedy of long repute.[17]

Across the land, however, brandy proved the constant curative. As a stimulant, Berncastle claimed, it was 'an absolute specific in snake poison, by overcoming the paralysed state of the heart and forcing it quickly to resume its natural action'.[18] With doses ranging from 'a nobbler' to several bottles, proof that it was neutralising the venom could be discerned by the absence of intoxicating symptoms. Neither teetotallers nor minors as young as two escaped; even dogs received a nip. Not all agreed, however. 'I cannot understand on what theory this idea of saturating with spirit every poor wretch, who is supposed to have been bitten by a snake is based', complained Creswick Hospital surgeon, John Webb, in 1872, 'yet it is the practice the public always adopt, whenever they can get a chance ... [and] not disapproved of by the majority of practitioners'.[19]

Berncastle's Victorian entrée coincided with a dead end in Halford's snakebite researches. Although in March 1868 he touted a customised a pair of scissors 'to cut out the piece, and throw away the poison', this sadistic-sounding implement did not catch on.[20] He therefore took a different tack. In Melbourne's *Argus* of 5 December 1867, 'George B. Halford' admitted to observing as snake showman Joseph Shires was bitten by a tiger snake, adding that Shires's Antidote saved its proprietor while the same serpent 'killed a dog and a kitten, both within one hour'.[21] A fortnight later, 'Professor Halford' reported that after bites by tiger snakes, only three of thirteen dogs treated with Shires's Antidote recovered, plus one of seven untreated animals. 'As regards the value of the antidote as a means of saving dogs', he noted, 'your readers are now as good judges as myself'.[22]

Halford, however, faced a different judgement. During the inquest into the death of Joseph Drummond in May 1868 (see Chapter 2), he disingenuously denied writing the first letter. At issue was not the dead dog or kitten, but his admission of experimenting upon Shires. That the pedlar chose to be bitten was beyond doubt. But in 1868, for a professor to endanger human life by encouraging a deliberate snakebite went beyond the pale. His authority threatened clinically, scientifically and legally, Halford needed to move forward. Attuned to escalating alarm over snakebite, but unable to experiment upon patients without public censure, the *Argus* incident affirmed that Victorians displayed no such squeamishness about his vivisections.

Dogs, dogma and dogmatism

Halford soon found a new direction, inspired by Silas Weir Mitchell's return to snakebite studies. Staggered by American medical credulity for proliferating 'cures', Mitchell asserted that 'the puzzling factor of individuality' and 'cases of unusual resistance' necessitated multiple experiments.[23] While every putative remedy failed Mitchell's vivisectional tests, by October 1868 Halford too was exploring a novel antidote: intravenous injection of ammonia. His critical first trial utilised not an Australian toxin, but rattlesnake venom supplied by Mitchell. Moribund within 24 hours, his canine subject was instantaneously revived by two injections of liquor ammoniæ fortissimus diluted in water. Treating another five dogs following bites or inoculation with tiger snake venom, Halford trumpeted that four survived to run about and eat heartily.[24]

In nineteenth-century experimental pathology, suggests William Bynum, it was 'altogether messier' to interpret animal models of injected poisons than inoculated pathogens.[25] Not so in Victoria. On 11 November, Beechworth surgeon John Dempster attended a patient bitten by a 'black snake'. The man kept sinking despite being treated 'in the usual way, with brandy and ammonia, and scarifying the wound and applying ammonia'. Having read of Halford's vivisections, the desperate rural doctor injected ammonia and the man immediately recovered. Fellow surgeon Alvara Slater and local Anglican rector W. Corbet Howard then experimented on several envenomed creatures; while ammoniacal injection 'roused the animals temporarily ... they all eventually succumbed'.[26] Thus, from the first, others' animal data could not confirm clinical claims made for Halford's method.

Undaunted, he sought to prove that his remedy was not innately poisonous by outlining a pair of 'painless vivisections' to the Medical Society of Victoria on 7 April 1869. Two dogs were chloroformed and their chest cavities opened. Repeated ammonia injections into their jugular veins dramatically increased the heart rate, rousing the thoracotomised beasts to full consciousness, necessitating further chloroform. After eight cycles the anguished animals were killed.[27]

Responding politically rather than morally, the anti-Halford *Australian Medical Gazette* hoped 'that the cruel and disgusting vivisections of the French school of experimenters, and of which the unfortunate canine race are the principal victims, will never be introduced into Victoria; indeed, we are very doubtful of the scientific value of "interrogating nature" in such a cruel and unnatural fashion'.[28] Against this patently hypocritical critique – given the *Gazette*'s regular support of Indian experimentalists like Fayrer – Halford's research hardly epitomised empirical or ethical rectitude. He began routinely experimenting upon animals, chirping that a putative anaesthetic enabled him to 'hack [a dog] about as I liked'.[29]

Indeed, Halford had a problematic relationship with hounds throughout his career. Insisting that both laity and doctors could replicate his techniques and results, he resisted the 'boundary and regulation work' corralling the coalescing discipline of experimental physiology.[30] Unlike European vivisectors, Halford revealed his techniques to the public. Seeking to multiply witnesses, he required readers to interpret his performances rather than physically visiting his laboratory.[31] As his trial of Shires's Antidote attested, the results were intended to speak for themselves.

What remained inconstant were Halford's homologies. In shaping modern Japan, asserts Aaron Skabelund, canines acted both physically and symbolically as 'brokers in human interactions'. Paraphrasing Gayatri Spivak to ask, 'Can the subaltern bark?', he contends that dogs were never silent historical actants.[32] Yet translating animal data into human bodies remained contentious throughout the nineteenth century.[33] The Victorian era, suggest Neil Pemberton and Michael Worboys, sustained a permeable boundary between human and veterinary medicine.[34] By mid-century Rudolf Virchow – Europe's master of cellular pathology – posited an underlying unity of animal and human health. Chris Degeling positions this gambit not as an epistemic moment, but the projection of a unifying 'disease-world' generated by biological laboratories.[35]

Aware of Virchow's philosophy, Halford saw canine and human outcomes converge: dogs were both his technologies and the potential beneficiaries of his snakebite antidote. But how did hounds and humans figure within his moral universe? As Harriet Ritvo suggests, emphasising human–canine homologies could defuse disturbing taxonomic and evolutionary questions regarding the animality of *Homo sapiens* vis-à-vis apes.[36] As a corollary of his 'gorilla warfare' of 1863–65 (see Chapter 3), elevating laboratory dogs in the order of creation furthered Halford's pietistic, political and pragmatic agendas.

This is not to impute a sentimental attachment to strays. However, it would be anachronistic to infer from late modern biomedicine that Halford was cognitively and emotionally detached from his dogs. Stephen Pemberton demonstrates how, even late into the twentieth century, the fragility of haemophiliac dogs overrode their ostensible fungibility as experimental objects, elevating their ethical status and impelling a 'necessity to care'.[37] Many nineteenth-century laboratories likewise fostered an intimate, almost veterinary, relationship between scientist and subject. This 'psychosocial sympathy between experimenters and canines' permitted investigators to read meaning from the gestures, behaviours and utterances of individual vivisectional subjects.[38] To answer both Skabelund and Spivak, Halford's dogs could 'speak'.

Clinical miracles and the retreat from animals

Halford soon found an opportunity to apply his remedy clinically. On 30 November 1868 he attended John Brown, a suburban stationmaster poisoned by a 'brown snake' and displaying the prototypical signs: lassitude, vomiting, progressive paralysis and 'coma'. Local surgeon George Arnold had employed excision, ligature, dousing with liquor ammoniæ fortissimus, oral administration of six ounces (175 ml) of brandy admixed with aromatic ammonia spirit, smelling salts, mustard poultices to the hands, feet and abdomen, galvanism and frogmarching.[39] His colleague William A'Beckett urged calling out Halford, who 'consented with some hesitancy' to inject ammonia 'as a last resort, inasmuch as the curative process, although proved by experiments on quadrupeds to be theoretically true, had not yet been practised on a human being'.[40] Brown's dramatic recovery convinced A'Beckett that Halford's technique saved the stationmaster, but the professor never injected it into another human.

Ammonia treatment for snakebite nevertheless accelerated across Victoria. Six successes were reported before 1868 ended, including unfortunate 14-year-old Isabella Mellross, bitten by a tiger snake on Christmas Eve and a black snake on Christmas Day.[41] But victories were counterbalanced by unpleasant sequelae: muscular spasms, choking, vomiting and sometimes panic verging on hysteria. Significant vein damage was a common, concerning and disfiguring side-effect, occasionally causing large sloughs.

Hyperbole, however, soon supplanted testimony. 'The name of Professor Halford', lauded a correspondent in Melbourne's *Economist*, 'will descend to posterity encircled with a halo of imperishable renown'.[42] When William Rae injected ammonia into a moribund patient outside his surgery, the assembled crowd expressed 'great astonishment at the immediate result'.[43] Respected surgeon Francis Laidlaw likewise enthused that 'people present in the room seemed perfectly astounded at such a result from the injection ... using the language of one who was present, "By God Sir, it was like magic"'.[44] Indeed, 'remarkable, 'wonderful', 'marvellous' and 'magical' proved a constant refrain. Its acme issued from surgeon John Lane, who extolled 'the almost Godlike power of Ammonia'.[45]

Such deification was not lost on practitioners competing with home remedies and patent nostrums. Halford urged caution, requesting that each case be observed and documented, writing personally to almost all clinicians who used his remedy. Charles Campbell agrees that intravenous ammonia was doubtless a potent stimulant, but whether it roused patients from the effects of snakebite or copious alcohol remains unclear. At this moment, he contends, Halford became 'whole-heartedly committed to a method of treatment no longer based on science'.[46] Amidst his expanding circle of clinical witnesses, humans superseded dogs as informants. What, therefore, constituted Halford's 'science' as 1869 ended?

Halford's syringe and his witness-participants

Unlike experimental physiology, argues Bruno Latour, the ascent of bacteriology required transposing laboratories to public arenas. For 'the new agent to do everything that the old disease did, the Pasteurians had to link it, in the most invincibly sceptical minds, with all the symptoms of the disease through spectacular experiments'.[47] Livestock – as victims of anthrax – became translation devices linking laboratory to field. But critically for Louis Pasteur, inoculating anthrax via syringe remained an artificial process; his crowds were convinced only when he transmitted anthrax bacillus to cows through 'natural' means: contaminated feed mixed with thistles.

Such manoeuvres were superfluous for snakebite investigators. First fashioned in the 1660s, the syringe and hypodermic needle long presented a theriomorphic conundrum: did it mimic a serpent's fang, or vice versa? Although affordable syringes only penetrated the Australian market in the 1860s, they rapidly emblematised both the measured envenomation of Halford's experimental animals and the calibrated delivery of his therapeutic. If this device soon became ubiquitous across the Australian colonies, animal experiments likewise escaped his laboratory. Halford touted syringes to widen not merely his audience, but his circle of witness-participants. Any settler, he claimed, could excise the bitten area and open a vein to introduce the needle. Indeed, Halford urged, 'practise the operation upon a dead dog or sheep … and afterwards get some friends to hold a live animal and repeat it', so that one 'need have no fear of doing the same thing to a living man'.[48]

Dogs, as much as humans, were beneficiaries. Colonists had long shared medicaments with their domesticates (Figure 18). If veterinarians remained unconvinced about injecting ammonia into canine veins, Victorians were not. Traversing Gippsland with the Geodetic Survey in 1870, Government Astronomer Robert Ellery used

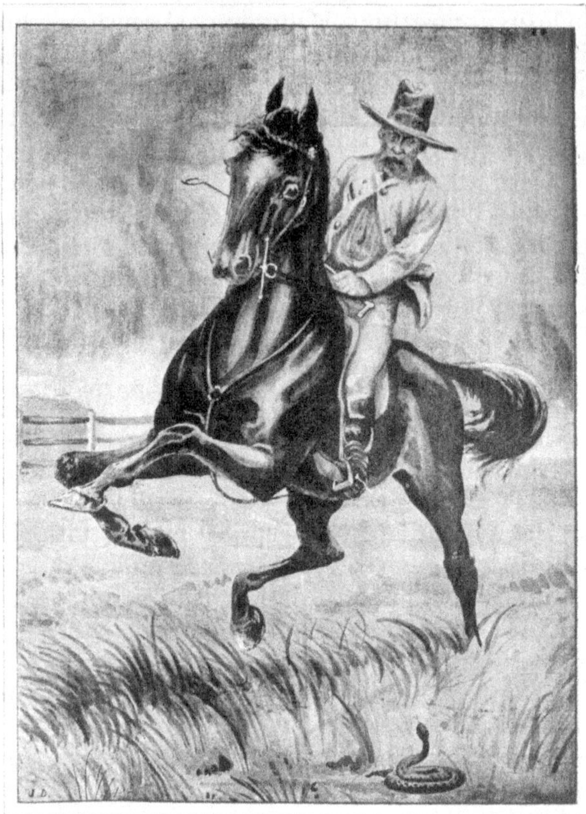

18 'A snake in the grass', *Illustrated Australian News*, 1 January 1891.

'one of the small injection-syringes and ammonia' to save a dog bitten by a tiger snake. By 1875, he remarked, injecting ammonia into snake-bitten beasts was so common that it was 'no more spoken of than the bleeding of a horse'.[49]

From 1870, kits comprising a syringe, ammonia and tweezers to lift the bitten part for excision were sold throughout the colonies (Figure 19). British immigrant Ada Cambridge's first purchase for her new rural life was 'Professor Halford's snake-bite cure ... in a neat pocket-case'.[50] Commanding the same price as Berncastle's snakebite tin, by 1872 doctors and chemists commonly endorsed 'Halford's syringe', pre-filled with half a drachm (~ 2 ml) of liquor ammoniæ in water, with dilutions varying from 1:2 to 1:5. 'So much attention has been given to ammonia injection and its magical effects by the press', warned prominent Melbourne surgeon Patrick Smith, 'the very syringe

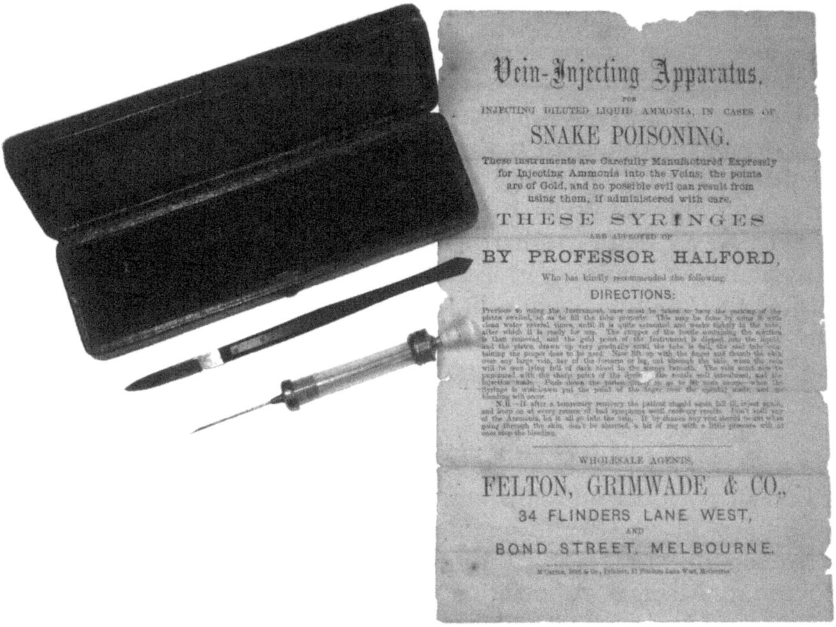
Vein-Injecting Apparatus,
INJECTING DILUTED LIQUID AMMONIA, IN CASES OF
SNAKE POISONING.
These Instruments are Carefully Manufactured Expressly for Injecting Ammonia into the Veins; the points are of Gold, and no possible evil can result from using them, if administered with care.
THESE SYRINGES
BY PROFESSOR HALFORD,
DIRECTIONS:
WHOLESALE AGENTS,
FELTON, GRIMWADE & CO.,
34 FLINDERS LANE WEST,
BOND STREET, MELBOURNE.

19 Kit for injecting ammonia for snakebite, comprising scalpel, syringe, instructions and case, *c.*1869.

(which to some is a token of a new triumph of science) so appeals to the love of the novel, and quasi-scientific, that it has come to be regarded by the bushman as the sole and only remedy'.[51]

Both ammonia and syringes embodied not merely an escalating colonial circulation of commodities, but what Arjun Appadurai has termed a 'traffic in criteria', the trade in expertise that nuances their 'technical, social and aesthetic appropriateness'.[52] While a pungent whiff of ammonia 'for snake bites and head-aches' formed the centrepiece of Stanley Morton's choreographed encounter with an East African warlord in 1871, no tournament of authentication ensued against the competing Arabic *dawa*.[53] Conversely, as Paul Foley and Luke Keogh have elaborated, western adoption of the Australian indigenous shrub pituri – a narcotic agent traded widely via Aboriginal exchange circuits – required multiple modes of verification in the 1870s to transform it into a viable commodity. These encompassed provenancing dried leaves to a living plant, observation of Aboriginal methods of preparation and consumption, chemical analysis, isolation of extracts, experimental testing upon dogs, cats and rats, and transnational transfer of samples to Paris, London and Edinburgh.[54] Credulity persisted, certainly, but the consumer landscape was changing.

Whether deployed for human or canine patients, the epistemological basis for the 'magical' recoveries following ammonia injection in Victoria was patent to all observers. Thus, like Pasteur, Halford's technique spectacularly verified his assertions. Unlike Pasteur, however, he encouraged others to multiply the experiment themselves, transplanting his treatment to wider terrains. Errors – especially spilling ammonia onto or under the skin – caused many debilitating side-effects. Nevertheless, in harried circumstances, the syringe promised a regularity of administration and a measured quantity of the remedy. Tested in Halford's hounds, practised in settlers' dogs and proven by their recovery when bitten by snakes, the animal origins of this practice remained at the heart of its widespread adoption.

A collective experiment?

Clinical, political and epistemological critiques of Halford and his technique all orbited the appropriate constitution of 'evidence'. They dominated – and perhaps motivated – the first meetings of the Victorian Medical Association from its establishment in January 1869. Berncastle urged members to lobby the Victorian government to enshrine his own approach as the approved treatment for snakebite and to officially discourage ammonia injection.[55] This edict did not eventuate. Concurrently the Association's official organ – the new *Australian Medical Gazette* – delighted in broadcasting failures of ammonia injection, likening Professor Halford to patent pill purveyor, 'Professor Holloway'.[56] Such critiques persisted – quite literally – until the *Gazette*'s final page in December 1871.

Halford consistently insisted that ammonia was not a 'specific' for snakebite. Rather, he theorised in 1869, injected ammonia stimulated 'the heart and the cells of the cerebral, spinal, and sympathetic ganglia, by which means the whole system, mental and corporeal, is roused into action'.[57] Anatomical variations, plus differential susceptibility to 'excitability', explained both clinical divergence between individuals and difficulties extrapolating results across species. Indeed, additional animal studies saw Halford return to haematology. 'In fatal cases of snake-poisoning, whether in this colony, India, America or Africa, the blood loses its power of coagulation, and becomes thinner and poorer', he explained. As 'a force communicated from without, potential in the syringe, active in the body', ammonia effected both central and peripheral stimulation: the heart pumped anew and the 'stagnating' blood circulated.[58]

Garlands proliferated. A large meeting of Melbourne's elite in March 1870 lauded his innovation and urged a public subscription to further

Halford's researches.[59] Elected President of the Medical Society of Victoria in January 1871, Halford was extolled by his predecessor as an eminent physiologist who 'clearly established, not only by physiological experiments upon animals, but by actual experience on man' the means to counteract snakebite and blood poisoning.[60] That May, when Parliamentarian Wilberforce Stephen conferred a handsome book of testimonials to 'the high sense which is entertained of the importance of his discovery', Halford outlined his credo:

> You shut an animal up in the same room as a snake. The snake bites it; presently you see it fall, and it dies. There is no obscurity about this – the cause of death is evident. You must watch all the symptoms of change in the animal's blood. You must work away with whole tribes of this creature, and so endeavour to master the problem. Once you have a clue to the mystery of blood-poisoning, then perhaps you will be able to enter combat with cheerfulness with this and other dreadful poisons.[61]

A motion was passed to lobby for funds permitting Halford 'to obtain specimens of the lower animals and the suitable appliances to enable him to make a series of experiments ... whereby some of the diseases most fatal to human life may be combated'.[62] Thus Victoria's elite sought state support for vivisection, if not a 'Government Anguinologist'. As Latour remarks of Pasteur's stratagems, once the 'capital of trust' invested in research programmes passes a critical point, doubt 'moves not in the direction of science but toward the inertia of public authorities'.[63]

As Halford's remedy came to embody the panacean hopes of fellow colonists, clear patterns emerged. In June 1870 he collated 20 reports of ammonia injection for snakebite; all but one arose from rural medical correspondents.[64] Two years later, with 30 cases recorded, support remained pointedly parochial: only one letter hailed from outside Victoria, rising to just four of 43 cases reported by 1875.[65] In Britain, nevertheless, both the *Medical Times and Gazette* and the *British Medical Journal* boosted Halford's research through the early 1870s. The latter suggested that Australian serpents were not only as deadly as the cobra and rattlesnake, but almost as venomous 'as some of his London critics'.[66] The *Lancet* of March 1870, for instance, berated Halford for 'gravely accepting a testimonial for having made two "discoveries", one of which is no discovery at all, and the other of which ranks among the oldest, most outstanding, and universally received methods of therapeutics'.[67] From *Nature* to the New York *Journal of Commerce*, the *Pall Mall Gazette* to *Punch*, the Atlantic world rendered Halford's ammonia injection between these extremes.[68]

As bluster succeeded hypothesis, Halford's diffuse network of Victorian witness-participants became his epistemology of proof. Clinical use of injected ammonia now comprised a collective experiment. By 1872 it was no longer a last resort: half of the snakebite cases reported that year employed Halford's technique 'at once'. Confident in this clinical verification, he could distance his science both from theory and from animal experimentation. It was precisely such human testimony that vivisectors in India vigorously contested.

Thanatophidia and therapeutics: ammonia injection in India

By November 1869 the *Medical Times and Gazette* acknowledged that Halford's 'plan of treatment is now well known here as elsewhere'.[69] Reading in mid-1870 that 'the action of the poison of your American snakes is similar to that of our Australian ones', *California Medical Gazette* subscribers were informed that ammonia injection was 'now recognised by the profession in Australia as a reliable cure'.[70] Several American physicians concurred, including James Knott of Atlanta, toasting 'Professor Halford, of Australia' for this 'magical treatment'.[71] In France, the prominent *Bulletin Général de Thérapeutique Médicale et Chirurgicale* translated one of Halford's lengthy articles, but within months declared his treatment worthless.[72]

India, as ever, remained the thorn in Halford's side. Although Pratik Chakrabarti proposes that sustained Indian research into snake venoms did not commence until the 1880s, in 1869 alone Joseph Fayrer enlisted over 100 domestic dogs, 'pariah dogs', fowls and pigeons to test a welter of venoms and remedies.[73] Initially admitting that 'ammonia may have been so far beneficial', his evidence soon suggested otherwise.[74] After injecting ammonia into 15 animals, just one fowl and two dogs survived – the only three creatures not envenomed. Hundreds of further animal experiments through 1870–71 only deepened Fayrer's pessimism towards ever finding a reliable snakebite cure.

Such negativity was not the prevailing mood, nor was vivisection the pre-eminent mode. 'The clinical evidence on record in favour of ammonia injections in snake-bite', opined the *British Medical Journal* in 1871, 'seems to us to outweigh the experimental failures of Dr. Fayrer.'[75] Puzzled that none 'of the hundreds of medical officers in India ... can accept Professor Halford's facts or theories, *so far as Indian snakes are concerned*', the *Medical Times and Gazette* challenged Halford to pit his method against cobra venom.[76]

Even on the subcontinent, Fayrer's results disappointed. In 1872 his magnum opus, *The Thanatophidia of India*, catalogued his venom studies since 1867. If its conclusions on the utility of antidotes proved convincingly nihilistic, Fayrer also said surprisingly little about the nature of venom. Nevertheless, he conceded that different venoms exhibited divergent effects on coagulation – at least in animals. In 1871 he forwarded cobra venom to the City and Guilds of London Institute for chemical analysis prior to physiological characterisation by Thomas Lauder Brunton, lecturer in materia medica and therapeutics at St Bartholomew's Hospital. Probably Britain's most eminent pharmacologist, Brunton's vivisections identified the alcohol-soluble fraction as the more fatal constituent, but refused to speculate on its toxicological mechanisms.[77]

Fayrer's conclusions on the nature of snake venom were thus predominantly observational, derived from signs exhibited by his hecatombs of experimental animals. 'Reading' their suffering, he surmised that venom produced 'fatal or deleterious effects, either by completely paralysing the nerve centres, and thus causing rapid dissolution, or by partially paralysing them, and poisoning the blood'.[78] His therapeutic pessimism was shared by fellow army surgeon Edward Nicholson, whose 1870 *Indian Snakes* asserted, 'if the snake has really injected poison into your system, unless you have the means of applying at once very active measures, you had best hang up your harp on the willow tree'.[79] On the subcontinent, approved methods mirrored those employed in Australia: ligature, scarification, suction, cautery, acid, exploding gunpowder in the bite, galvanism and freely imbibing liquor ammoniæ mixed with water, hot brandy, rum or whisky. Although Halford's injection seemed 'more rational than most suggestions that have been made', Fayrer lamented, 'I regret exceedingly that in my own experiments it has proved of no avail'.[80]

Challengers near and far

Initially, metropolitan opinion largely upheld Halford's credibility. In the *Medical Times and Gazette*, he likened studying snakebite to toxicologists testing prussic acid or pathologists scrutinising syphilis: it afforded 'unmistakable evidence of direct inoculation or infection, and present[ed] a series of results directly flowing therefrom'.[81] He hypothesised that ammonia chemically reoxygenated blood, whilst directly stimulating cardiac nerve filaments to effect arterial dilation, enhanced circulation, bodily warming and a slow but steady heart rhythm. Citing recent neurophysiological studies to argue that differing spinal and ganglionic anatomy accounted for the variable effects of snakebite in dogs and humans, Halford aimed to undermine the pillars of Fayrer's authority: his unifying neurotoxic theory and his diversity of experimental animals. Indeed, Halford 'urged upon the medical men of India to try injecting ammonia into the veins of men, even if they have failed of success with dogs'.[82]

Halford's gambit intersected with Fayrer's nihilism: by 1872 Indian clinicians commenced testing ammonia injection. In demonstrating the inutility of ammonia injection for Indian snakebites, however, their cases furthermore promulgated an intercolonial rivalry, belittling Australian venoms as lacklustre. Even Fayrer's experiments forced him to admit that 'quantity for quantity, the poisons of different genera, even species, vary considerably'.[83] This belated concession concurred with North Carolina homeopath Sylvester Higgins, whose 1873 monograph *Ophidians* asserted that insisting upon a single venom uniting all serpents was 'quite contrary to the experience of every person who has had to cure many cases of snake-bite'.[84]

Fayrer was, moreover, far from Halford's most strident critic. In June 1873 Balasore civil surgeon Vincent Richards lambasted Halford's weak evidence for ammonia injection, asserting it 'quite possible that some fallacy underlies his experiments on the lower animals'.[85] Commencing his own vivisections, Richards offered cobra venom to Halford, requesting that Australian snake poisons be sent to Fayrer – now in London – or Joseph Ewart, Professor of Physiology at the Calcutta Medical College. Ignoring this request, as he had snubbed Mitchell in 1868, Halford was now circumvented. In July 1873, Fayrer enlisted Richards, Ewart and Stephen Coull Mackenzie – Professor of Hygiene at Calcutta Medical College – to join a Government of India commission investigating 'the effects of artificial respiration, intravenous injection of ammonia, and administration of various drugs, &c. in Indian and Australian snake-poisoning'.[86] Acknowledging the divergent results of Fayrer and Halford's investigations, Ewart lobbied both the Surgeon-General and the Lieutenant-Governor of Bengal, whose entreaties to the Victorian Government saw twelve tiger snakes and another dozen red-bellied black snakes transhipped to Calcutta in February 1874. As an act of 'animal diplomacy', however, it constituted a flawed gesture: neither donor nor recipient accumulated prestige or popularity via the translocation of these 'dangerous' Australian beasts.[87]

This Indian-Australian contest proved purely vivisectional; although 'ferocious', none of the imported ophidians bit an Indian investigator. Perhaps responding to criticisms of Fayrer's diversity of experimental animals, dogs were used exclusively. But they were not mere dogs. In testing artificial respiration, each canine was hybridised with a manually operated bellows, connected via India-rubber tubing to a cannula inserted into its trachea. Adding hypodermic syringes, the Commission's dogs thus became the most highly instrumented creatures hitherto employed for snakebite studies. It did little for their moral status. Any intimacy Halford may have shared with his canine subjects receded with each Indian experiment. Neither the dogs' distress, nor their individual resilience, counted. They were simply abstract instruments deprived of volition; even their 'frequent vomiting and defæcation as early symptoms of poisoning, [and] excessive flow of urine and saliva later on [indicated] an attempt on the part of *nature* to eliminate the poison from the body'.[88]

The Indian Snakebite Commission excoriated Halford, his Victorian colleagues and their patients for lacking 'that scientific precision and accurate observation of facts which alone must be allowed to carry conviction'. Even the transplanted serpents were criticised. Each yielded under two grains (130 mg) of venom, whilst the cobra's flood of 13 grains (845 mg) was decreed 'more powerful and mortal' than either Australian venom.[89] The Commissioners castigated Halford for suggesting that antipodean snakebites were as deadly as cobra bites in dogs or – by implication – humans. Omitting to mention that, dose-for-dose, tiger snake and cobra venom had proved equally deadly, they insisted that cobras were 'six to thirteen times more poisonous than the snakes of Australia'.[90]

Dolefully, the Commissioners concluded from their vivisections that artificial respiration only forestalled expiry after envenomation, while intravenous injection of ammonia conclusively hastened death. Yet no Australian, Indian or British pundit questioned whether the dogs themselves were identical across Imperial contexts. This unitarian insistence in the face of canine morphological diversity was curious given nineteenth-century obsessions with pedigrees, exacerbated by ongoing colonial tensions over atavistic interbreeding with 'savage' indigenous pariah dogs, wolves and dingoes.[91]

The collapse of clinical testimony

Although Fayrer uncharacteristically deemed the Indian Snakebite Commission's recommendations 'encouraging', none saved lives. 'This was not at all a satisfactory experiment', he reiterated, and Indian colleagues concurred.[92] If Edward Nicholson declined to vivisect, professing 'a great dislike to anything like cruelty to animals', in the 1874 edition of *Indian Snakes* he propounded a Darwinian regionalism founded on anatomy rather than physiology. Inefficient injection of venom through the short fangs of Australian serpents, he suggested, explained why 'moribund persons rise at once, walk and eat' following ammonia injections.[93]

Halford stood firm. By 1874 his local correspondents reported 32 cases, nearly 80% successful. As ever, humans were not the sole beneficiaries. Rescuing a 'fine greyhound', Geelong surgeon David Stoddart evoked its testimony: 'when I spoke to the dog by name, it wagged its tail'.[94] On 27 August, MP John Madden lobbied Victoria's Legislative Assembly for £500 to aid Halford's research into ammonia injection for snakebite and blood-poisoning. When the motion passed, the *Argus* added that he 'would probably have been "decorated" before now' had he 'rendered similar services to the state in England, India, or on the Continent of Europe'.[95] Yet after the Indian Commission, Europeans increasingly distanced themselves from Melbourne's professor. Asserting that Australian snakebites were trifling, the formerly loyal *British Medical Journal* likened antipodean doctors to 'Hindoos' for blindly employing antidotes 'shown by exact experiments to be valueless'.[96] Thus was the animal matrix layered across multiple sites of empire.

Amidst these Imperial divisions, on 17 March 1875 the Medical Society of Victoria convened to adjudicate on Halford's method. The 'cases and opinions previously recorded here have been discredited', complained President (Thomas) Aubrey Bowen, 'both by the Government commission in India and by the leading medical journal in England'. Insisting that 'every old resident in the bush of this country can relate cases of horses, cattle, and dogs killed by snakes', he yet urged members to be 'very cautious in forming conclusive deductions as to the effects of remedies on human beings from experiments performed on animals'.[97]

Melbourne's medical elite upheld their honour with human cases. Bowen and Halford detailed 43 ammonia injections for snakebite, a 70-page catalogue filling the entire March 1875 issue of the *Australian Medical Journal*. Listing just three fatal outcomes (6.9%), their message was clear: practitioner experience trumped animal data. Their gambit, however, faltered. William McCrea – Chairman of Victoria's Central Board of Health since 1853 – proposed countering the Indian Commission's claims by replicating their experiments, because prior Victorian trials lacked 'the same scientific accuracy'.[98] Halford was outraged. Recapitulating that his laboratory had been 'pretty well strewed with dead dogs during these experiments', his acme of proof comprised the clinical reports of 'highly-qualified medical gentlemen'.[99]

When he stormed out, the meeting nevertheless appointed a subcommittee to undertake animal experiments testing ammonia injection. Although Halford supporter William Gillbee insisted that snakebite studies were 'emphatically a Government duty', the Society contributed £25, prompting the colony's Chief Secretary to superadd £50 to Parliament's £500 award.[100] Further imbricating vivisection into Victoria's institutional edifice, experimental work was largely conducted at the Richmond Police Depôt, employing tiger snakes delivered via the Swan Hill police station.[101] Led first by McCrea and then senior surgeon Tharp Girdlestone, between 3 February and 13 April 1876 the experimenters injected venom subcutaneously into over 60 dogs, forcing snakes to directly bite another 14 strays and one small goat.

The results spoke volumes. Regardless of treatment, no dog recovered from more than half a grain (~ 30 mg) of venom. The pitiful sequelae included vomiting, progressive paralysis, laboured breathing, pupillary dilation, convulsions, insensibility, then apnoeic death. Given that most dogs became patently distressed after envenomation, ammonia injection must have been remarkably unpleasant for the subcommittee to single out its adverse effects. One dog's 'great pain' and howling showed that the poor beast 'evidently suffered' from leakage of ammonia at the injection site. While it died, another animal surviving a small venom dose developed such a large, painful ammonia slough that it was put down.[102]

Indeed, the Victorian experimenters grew increasingly sensitive to their dogs' suffering. When Halford was invited to inject his remedy, it was noteworthy that the creature 'did *not* struggle or howl on the injection of ammonia'.[103] Whether from moral sensitivity or the clinical implications, the subcommittee could no longer avoid the painful truth. Ammonia injection caused not just swelling, vomiting and convulsions, but sometimes proved more rapidly fatal than snakebite. 'The results in our own and the Indian experiments have been so uniform', observed one investigator, 'as almost to resemble experiments in physics and chemistry.'[104] 'The Society had before it a serious responsibility', McCrea pinpointed. 'It had to decide between the cases reported to Professor Halford, and the experiments now recorded by the committee.'[105]

'Confined to mongrels?'

This question vexed the Medical Society of Victoria. Thomas Fitzgerald – Melbourne University's lecturer in surgery – was blunt: did any of the investigators profess clinical experience with injecting ammonia, 'or was it all confined to mongrels?'[106] Henry Wooldridge, present when Halford had treated stationmaster John Brown in January 1869, concurred. 'One good fact obtained by actual practice in man, is worth a thousand experiments in dogs.'[107] But Girdlestone, as the subcommittee's chief experimentalist, declared the canine results unquestionable and of direct human relevance. Indeed, clinical reports of 'miraculous' recoveries now mitigated against their verisimilitude.[108] McCrea – another former Halford ally – warned that injecting ammonia after snakebite now amounted to 'trifling with human life'.[109]

Faced with animal data and apostate champions, Halford accepted the subcommittee's vivisections but insisted that 'experiments had gone beyond dogs, and we had evidence much more conclusive than they could afford'.[110] The impasse was debated through successive meetings until a formal motion coalesced to resolve the three issues dividing the profession since 1868:

1. That the bites of Australian poisonous snakes are extremely deadly.
2. That the symptoms are the same in Australia as in India; that they differ somewhat in animals and man; that they are distinct in character from those of alcoholism.
3. That ammonia is the best form of stimulant to exhibit, and that the intra-venous injection is the best method for its administration.[111]

Ambushing voters at the July meeting, McCrea summarised a questionnaire that he, as Chief Medical Officer, had hastily circulated to 95 Victorian practitioners. His flawed data purported to show that ammonia treatment drastically increased mortality: of 40 snakebitten patients receiving Halford's injection, 15 (37.5%) died, versus 6 deaths (2.8%) among 211 patients treated otherwise.[112] Nevertheless, on 5 July 1876 the Medical Society of Victoria voted to override their own experimental subcommittee's report, formally adopting Halford's ammonia injection as their approved treatment for snakebite.

The elite, however, did not prevail. Although patients continued to receive Halford's remedy, reports steadily grew askance. Calumniating from Bengal, even Richards admitted to injecting ammonia into an Indian bitten by a cobra – with nugatory effect.[113] In November 1876, an exasperated *Lancet* demanded it was 'surely time that we heard the last of this subject'.[114] It was. Thereafter, Halford experimented rarely and published little. Throughout the following decade, snakebite reports drastically receded across Australia (Figure 20). If few employed Halford's method, fewer experimented with alternatives. By 1883 physician Ernest Wuth complained to the Medical Society of Victoria of 'a most lamentable want of progress' in local snakebite research.[115]

Yet the tail of Halford's technique remained long. In 1885 Richards fumed that ammonia injection was 'still to be found recommended in the pages of some of our standard works'; it resided in the authoritative Martindale's *Pharmacopœia* until 1910, the year of Halford's death.[116] With Australian snake charmers and senior physicians alike still swearing by ammonia injection into World War I, Halford was praised as a champion of the hypodermic syringe in Fielding Garrison's oft-reprinted

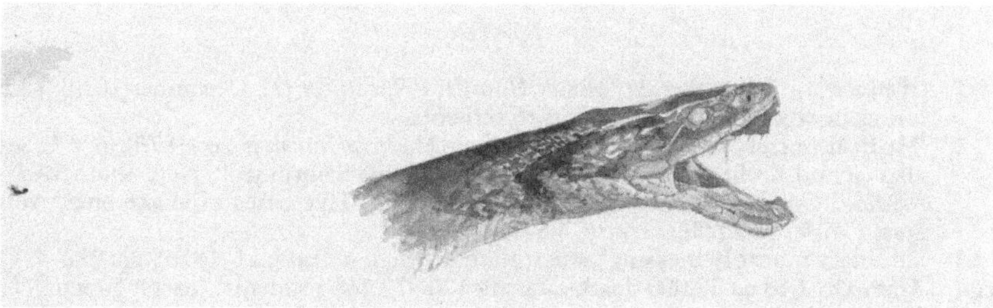

20 A.P. Marten, 'Brown snake that killed black boy on our plantation [Pleystowe, Queensland]', January 1875.

Introduction to the History of Medicine.[117] Indeed, from 1868 to 1875, Halford's colony of witness-participants had enrolled patients in what might now be loosely labelled a 'clinical trial'. Embracing the syringe, Victorian practitioners experimented with injecting liquor ammoniæ, ergotin and milk into patients for conditions ranging from scarlatina to typhoid fever. What colonial doctors increasingly demanded, however, was a measured mode of treatment, a cogent scientific rationale and 'proof' generated in experimental animals.

In this regard, 1876 proved doubly significant. Just a week before their definitive vote against animal data, the Medical Society of Victoria heard that Britain's premier physiologists considered extrapolations from dogs to humans eminently reasonable.[118] Indeed, while reining in British experimental practice, the Royal Commission on Vivisection admitted 'no possibility of arriving at any knowledge of an antidote for snake bite ... except by submitting animals to be bitten by snakes'.[119] Yet their gaze focused solely on India. Staggeringly, the Commissioners overlooked the profound epistemological schisms over the role and meaning of animal experiments that had publicly and acrimoniously divided antipodean and subcontinental venom investigators for a decade.[120]

This convergence prompts a critical question: Where was the moral dimension to the protracted Victorian–Indian exchanges? Unlike Britain, where vivisectors studied disease agents that were rarely 'seen', in the colonies – as Halford attested – there was no obscurity to snakebite. Whether canines benefited or suffered from his technique, what was being effaced over 1868–76 was the value of experimental creatures as individual subjects. Their integration with devices – from India-rubber tubing to hypodermic needles – increasingly rendered animals as objects. Dogs sank lower than a snake's belly within this matrix of moral hierarchies, yet, whether wagging a tail or howling in pain, they spoke.

Notes

1 'Wednesday, December 21, 1870', *Hamilton Spectator* (21 December 1870), p. 2. Italics in original; 'anguine' refers to serpents.
2 'Medical Society of Victoria', *Australian Medical Journal*, 20 (1875), p. 67. See also Gerard Krefft, 'The order of snakes – ophidia (continued)', *New South Wales Medical Gazette*, 4:3 (1873), p. 77; F.H. Woods, 'Five cases of snake-bite', *New South Wales Medical Gazette*, 4:5 (1874), p. 131.
3 'Ordinary monthly meeting', *Australian Medical Journal*, 11 (1876), pp. 232–4.
4 Approximated as 20,000 deaths among 120,972,263 residents: Joseph Fayrer, *The Thanatophidia of India. Being a Description of the Venomous Snakes of the Indian Peninsula, With an Account of the Influence of Their Poison on Life and a Series of Experiments* (London: J. and A. Churchill, 1872), pp. 31–2.
5 Pratik Chakrabarti, *Bacteriology in British India: Laboratory Medicine and the Tropics* (Rochester: University of Rochester Press, 2012), p. 126.
6 M. Worboys, 'British colonial medicine and tropical imperialism: a comparative perspective', in A.M. Luyendijk-Elshout *et al.* (eds), *Dutch Medicine in the Malay Archipelago, 1816–1942* (Amsterdam: Rodopi, 1989), p. 165.
7 Barbara J. Hawgood, 'The life and viper of Dr Patrick Russell MD FRS (1727–1805): physician and naturalist', *Toxicon*, 32:11 (1994), p. 1300.
8 Albert C.L.G. Günther, *The Reptiles of British India* (London: Robert Hardwicke, 1864), pp. 167–8.
9 For instance, Gerard Krefft, *The Snakes of Australia; An Illustrated and Descriptive Catalogue of All the Known Species* (Sydney: Thomas Richards, 1869), pp. 46, 57.
10 Gerard Krefft, 'Descriptions of new Australian snakes', *Proceedings of the Zoological Society of London* (1869), p. 54.
11 See Khiun Liew, 'Making health public: English language newspapers and the medical sciences in colonial Malaya (1840s–1941)', *East Asian Science, Technology and Society*, 3:2–3 (2009), pp. 226–7.
12 John Harley Warner, 'The idea of science in English medicine: the "decline of science" and the rhetoric of reform, 1815–45', in Roger French and Andrew Wear (eds), *British Medicine in an Age of Reform* (London: Routledge, 1991), pp. 154–5.
13 T.S. Pensabene, *The Rise of the Medical Practitioner in Victoria* (Canberra: Australian National University, 1980), p. 177.
14 Susan Hardy, 'Ferments, zymes and the west wind: adapting disease theories and therapies in New South Wales, 1860–1880', in Harold Attwood and Geoffrey Kenny (eds), *Reflections on Medical History and Health in Australia: Third National Conference on Medical History and Health in Australia 1986* (Melbourne: Medical History Unit, University of Melbourne, 1987), p. 44; A.J. Proust, 'Medical care in the colony', in A.J. Proust (ed.), *A Social and Cultural History of Medicine in New South Wales in the 19*th *Century: Southern Tablelands and Monaro* (Forrest: A.J. Proust, 1999), pp. 39–40, 54–7.
15 Dr Berncastle, *Australian Snake Bites: Their Treatment and Cure. The Use and Abuse of Tobacco* (Melbourne: Mason Firth & Co., 1868), p. 5.
16 W.J. Moore, 'A case of snake-bite', *Indian Medical Gazette*, 3 (1868), p. 104.
17 Sharon Louise Wallace, 'Treatment of snakebite from Halford to Sutherland' (BMedSci thesis, University of Melbourne, 1983), pp. 69–78.
18 Berncastle, *Australian Snake Bites*, p. 8.
19 John H. Webb, 'Treatment of snake-bite', *Australian Medical Journal*, 17 (1872), p. 156.
20 George B. Halford, 'On a pair of scissors for the excision of snake-bite', *Transactions and Proceedings of the Royal Society of Victoria*, 9 (1868), p. 47.
21 George B. Halford, 'Shires's antidote for snake-bite', *Argus* (5 December 1867), p. 6.
22 George B. Halford, 'Professor Halford's experiments with Shires' antidote', *Argus* (20 December 1867), p. 6.

23 S.W. Mitchell, 'Experimental contributions to the toxicology of rattle-snake venom', *New York Medical Journal*, 6:4 (1868), pp. 292, 315–16.
24 George B. Halford, 'Professor Halford's experiment on snake-poisoning', *Argus* (7 November 1868), p. 6.
25 W.F. Bynum, '"C'est un malade": animal models and concepts of human diseases', *Journal of the History of Medicine and Allied Sciences*, 45:3 (1990), p. 409.
26 University of Melbourne Archives, Melbourne (hereafter UMA), 1981.0062, Halford, George Britton, 'Letters to Professor G. Halford referring to his antidote – injection with ammonia', 1867–1937, John Dempster to George Halford, 15 November 1868.
27 George B. Halford, *On the Injection of Ammonia Into the Circulation* (Melbourne: Stillwell and Knight, 1869), pp. 6–7.
28 'The Medical Society and Dr. Halford's treatment of snake-bites', *Australian Medical Gazette*, 1 (1869), p. 76.
29 George B. Halford, 'Further observations on the injection of remedies into the blood', *Australian Medical Journal*, 14 (1869), p. 337.
30 Peter Keating, Alberto Cambrosio, and Michael Mackenzie, 'The tools of the discipline: standards, models, and measures in the affinity/avidity controversy in immunology', in Adele E. Clarke and Joan H. Fujimura (eds), *The Right Tools for the Job: At Work in Twentieth-Century Life Sciences* (Princeton: Princeton University Press, 1992), p. 315.
31 See Steven Shapin and Simon Schaffer, *Leviathan and the Air Pump: Hobbes, Boyle, and the Experimental Life* (Princeton: Princeton University Press, 2011), p. 25.
32 Aaron Herald Skabelund, *Empire of Dogs: Canines, Japan, and the Making of the Modern World* (Ithaca: Cornell University Press, 2011), pp. 7, 14.
33 José Ramón Bertomeu-Sánchez, 'Popularizing controversial science: a popular treatise on poisons by Mateu Orfila (1818)', *Medical History*, 53:3 (2009), pp. 365–9.
34 Neil Pemberton and Michael Worboys, *Mad Dogs and Englishmen: Rabies in Britain, 1830–2000* (Houndmills: Palgrave Macmillan, 2007), p. 4.
35 Chris Degeling, 'Canines, consanguinity, and one-medicine: all the qualities of a dog except loyalty', *Health and History*, 10:2 (2008), pp. 23–4, 31. See also Bynum, '"C'est un malade"', pp. 401–13; Cheryl A. Logan, 'Before there were standards: the role of test animals in the production of empirical generality in physiology', *Journal of the History of Biology*, 35:2 (2002), pp. 345–8, 354–6.
36 Harriet Ritvo, 'Animal consciousness: some historical perspective', *American Zoologist*, 40:6 (2000), p. 849.
37 Stephen Pemberton, 'Canine technologies, model patients: the historical production of hemophiliac dogs in American biomedicine', in Susan Schrepfer and Philip Scranton (eds), *Industrializing Organisms: Introducing Evolutionary History* (New York: Routledge, 2004), pp. 202–5.
38 Degeling, 'Canines, consanguinity, and one-medicine', p. 31.
39 UMA 1981.0062 Letters to Professor G. Halford referring to his antidote, GJ Arnold to Professor Halford, 4 December 1868; George B. Halford, 'Injection of ammonia in snake poisoning', *Australian Medical Journal*, 13 (1868), pp. 390–1.
40 'Remarkable case of snake-bite at Elsternwick', *Age* (2 December 1868), p. 3.
41 UMA 1981.0062, Henry Barrett to George Halford, 28 December 1868.
42 UMA 1981.0062, Halford, George Britton, 'Newspaper cuttings relating to snake-bite and antidote i.e. ammonia (Prof G.B. Halford)', 1867–1876, letter from John Smith, *Economist*, 19 August 1869, n.p.
43 George B. Halford, 'Snake-poisoning and its treatment (continued)', *Medical Times and Gazette*, 2 (new series 57) (1873), p. 576.
44 'Medical Society of Victoria', p. 108.
45 J.P. Lane, 'A case of snake-poisoning', *Australian Medical Journal*, 15 (1870), p. 60.
46 C.H. Campbell, 'Professor Halford's new treatment of snake bite with the injection of ammonia into the veins', *Medical Journal of Australia*, 1 (1966), p. 1011.

47 Bruno Latour, *The Pasteurization of France*, trans. Alan Sheridan and John Law (Cambridge, Mass.: Harvard University Press, 1988), p. 76.
48 G.B. Halford, 'The remedy of snake-bite', *Argus* (30 January 1869), p. 6.
49 'Medical Society of Victoria', pp. 73–4.
50 Ada Cambridge, '(Arriving in Melbourne)', in Elizabeth Webby (ed.), *Colonial Voices: Letters, Diaries, Journalism and Other Accounts of Nineteenth-Century Australia* (St Lucia: University of Queensland Press, 1989), p. 47.
51 'Medical Society of Victoria', *Australian Medical Journal*, 21 (1876), p. 226.
52 Arjun Appadurai, 'Introduction: commodities and the politics of value', in Arjun Appadurai (ed.), *The Social Life of Things: Commodities in Cultural Perspective* (Cambridge: Cambridge University Press, 1986), p. 54.
53 Henry M. Stanley, *How I Found Livingstone: Travels, Adventures and Discoveries in Central Africa: Including an Account of Four Months' Residence with Dr. Livingstone* (London: Samson Low, Marston, Low, and Searle, 1872), pp. 333–5.
54 Paul Foley, '*Duboisia myoporoides*: the medical career of a native Australian plant', *Historical Records of Australian Science*, 17:1 (2006), pp. 37–45; Luke Keogh, '*Duboisia pituri*: a natural history', *Historical Records of Australian Science*, 22:2 (2011), pp. 199–214.
55 'Proceedings of the Victorian Medical Association', *Australian Medical Gazette*, 1 (1869), pp. 55–6.
56 For instance, 'Death from snake-bite after injection of ammonia into the veins', *Australian Medical Gazette*, 1 (1869), p. 49.
57 Halford, *On the Injection of Ammonia Into the Circulation*, p. 7.
58 George B. Halford, 'The treatment of snake-bite in Victoria', *Australian Medical Journal*, 15 (1870), pp. 165, 169–70.
59 'Local topics', *Australian Medical Journal*, 15 (1870), p. 95.
60 Hermann Jonasson, *Valedictory Address: The President of the Medical Society of Victoria for the Year 1870* (Melbourne: Stillwell and Knight, 1871), p. 4.
61 'Presentation of the Halford Testimonial', *Argus* (16 May 1871), p. 7.
62 *Ibid.*
63 Latour, *The Pasteurization of France*, p. 53.
64 Halford, 'The treatment of snake-bite in Victoria', p. 172.
65 Wallace, 'Treatment of snakebite from Halford to Sutherland', p. 41.
66 'The ammonia cure for snake-bite', *British Medical Journal*, 2:504 (1870), p. 224.
67 'Discoveries at Melbourne', *Lancet*, 95:2430 (1870), p. 456.
68 UMA 1981.0062, *passim*.
69 [Untitled], *Medical Times and Gazette*, 39 (1869), p. 616.
70 E.H. Hall, 'Professor Halford's treatment of snake bite by the injection of liquid ammonia into the veins', *California Medical Gazette*, 2 (1870), p. 229.
71 J.J. Knott, 'A case of rattlesnake bite successfully treated by injections of carbonate of ammonia into veins', *Medical and Surgical Reporter*, 37:1064 (1877), p. 47.
72 George B. Halford, 'Du traitement des morsures de serpents venimeux par les injections intra-veineuses d'ammoniaque', *Bulletin Général de Thérapeutique Médicale et Chirurgicale*, 88 (1874), pp. 258–71; Le Roy de Mericourt, 'Du traitement des morsures des serpents venimeux de l'Inde et de l'Australie par l'ammoniaque', *Bulletin Général de Thérapeutique Médicale et Chirurgicale*, 87 (1874), p. 362.
73 Chakrabarti, *Bacteriology in British India*, p. 119.
74 J. Fayrer, 'On the action of the cobra poison (continued)', *Edinburgh Medical Journal*, 15 (part II) (1870), p. 624.
75 'Ammonia injection for snake-bite', *British Medical Journal*, 1:540 (1871), p. 482.
76 'Professor Halford's treatment of snake-bites', *Medical Times and Gazette*, 1 (1873), pp. 445–6. Italics in original.
77 Fayrer, *The Thanatophidia of India* (first edition), pp. 150–1.
78 *Ibid.*, p. 37.
79 Edward Nicholson, *Indian Snakes. An Elementary Treatise on Ophiology with a*

Descriptive Catalogue of the Snakes Found in India and the Adjoining Countries (Madras: Higginbotham & Co., 1870), p. 39.

80 Fayrer, *The Thanatophidia of India* (first edition), p. 39.

81 George B. Halford, 'Snake-poisoning and its treatment', *Medical Times and Gazette*, 2 (new series 47) (1873), p. 90.

82 George B. Halford, 'Snake-poisoning and its treatment (continued)', p. 323.

83 Fayrer, *The Thanatophidia of India* (first edition), pp. 1–2, 14, 17.

84 S.B. Higgins, *Ophidians, Zoological Arrangement of the Different Genera, Including Varieties Known in North and South America, the East Indies, South Africa and Australia* (New York: Boericke & Tafel, 1873), p. 115.

85 Vincent Richards, 'The treatment of snake-bite by intravenous injection of ammonia. Letter from Mr. Vincent Richards', *Medical Times and Gazette*, I (1873), p. 639.

86 Joseph Ewart, Vincent Richards, and S. Coull Mackenzie, *Report on the Effects of Artificial Respiration, Intravenous Injection of Ammonia and Administration of Various Drugs, &c., in Indian and Australian Snake-Poisoning; and the Physiological, Chemical, and Microscopical Nature of Snake Poisons. By the Commission Appointed to Investigate the Subject* (Calcutta: Bengal Secretariat Press, 1874), p. 17.

87 See Nancy Cushing and Kevin Markwell, 'Platypus diplomacy: animal gifts in international relations', *Journal of Australian Studies*, 33:3 (2009), pp. 255–8.

88 Ewart, Richards and Mackenzie, *Report on the Effects of Artificial Respiration*, p. 6. Italics mine.

89 *Ibid.*, pp. 27–9.

90 'Snake poisoning', *Indian Medical Gazette*, 9:11 (1874), p. 303.

91 See for example Harriet Ritvo, 'Ordering creation, or maybe not', in Helen Small and Trudi Tate (eds), *Literature, Science, Psychoanalysis, 1830–1970: Essays in Honour of Gillian Beer* (Oxford: Oxford University Press, 2003), pp. 55–8.

92 J. Fayrer, 'Snake-poisoning in India (continued)', *Medical Times and Gazette*, 2 (new series 47) (1873), p. 492.

93 Edward Nicholson, *Indian Snakes. An Elementary Treatise on Ophiology with a Descriptive Catalogue of the Snakes Found in India and the Adjoining Countries*, 2nd edn (Madras: Higginbotham and Co., 1874), pp. 150, 153.

94 'Ammonia in snake-bites', *British Medical Journal*, 2:712 (1874), p. 256.

95 'Monday, August 31, 1874', *Argus* (31 August 1874), p. 4.

96 'Snake-poisoning in Australia', *British Medical Journal*, 2:758 (1875), p. 63.

97 'Medical Society of Victoria', pp. 66, 68–9.

98 *Ibid.*, pp. 131–2.

99 G.B. Halford, 'The Indian Commission on Snake-Poisoning', *Melbourne Medical Record*, 4 (1875), p. 4.

100 W. McCrea *et al.*, 'Report of the special committee on the subject of snake-poisoning', *Australian Medical Journal*, 21 (1876), p. 105.

101 Ann Tovell Archives, Brownless Biomedical Library, University of Melbourne, Melbourne, Vouchers in the experiments in snake-poisoning, 1876.

102 McCrea *et al.*, 'Report of the special committee on the subject of snake-poisoning', p. 120.

103 *Ibid.*, p. 125. Emphasis mine.

104 'Medical Society of Victoria', p. 226.

105 'Report of the special committee on snake-poisoning', *Australian Medical Journal*, 21 (1876), p. 153.

106 'Medical Society of Victoria', p. 220.

107 'The report of the special committee on the treatment of snake-poisoning', *Australian Medical Journal*, 21 (1876), p. 189.

108 'Resumed discussion upon the report of the snake-poisoning experiments committee', *Australian Medical Journal*, 21 (1876), p. 135.

109 'Medical Society of Victoria', p. 228.

110 'Resumption of the discussion on the report of the special committee on snake-poisoning', *Australian Medical Journal*, 21 (1876), p. 156.

111 'Medical Society of Victoria', p. 219.

112 'Ordinary monthly meeting', pp. 232–4. In particular, McCrea neglected to mention that in many cases ammonia had been applied as a last resort, and thus its use would naturally have been concentrated towards the moribund end of the spectrum.

113 Vincent Richards, 'A fatal case of snake bite; intravenous injection of ammonia; remarks on the application of the ligature in snake bite', *Indian Medical Gazette*, 11:12 (1876), p. 321.

114 'The ammonia treatment of snake-poisoning', *Lancet*, 108:2776 (1876), p. 695.

115 E.M. Wuth, 'A suggestion as to the modern treatment of snake poisoning', *Australian Medical Journal*, 5 (1883), p. 60.

116 Vincent Richards, *The Land-Marks of Snake-Poison Literature, Being a Review of the More Important Researches Into the Nature of Snake-Poisons*, 2nd edn (Calcutta: D.M. Traill, 1885), p. 162; W. Harrison Martindale and W. Wynn Westcott, *The Extra Pharmacopœia of Martindale and Westcott*, 14th edn (London: H.K. Lewis, 1910), p. 120.

117 'Ammonia and snakebite', *Chemist and Druggist of Australasia*, 10:7 (1895), p. 140; E. Florance, 'Snake bite', *Australasian Medical Gazette*, 31 (1912), pp. 56–7; Fielding H. Garrison, *An Introduction to the History of Medicine, with Medical Chronology, Suggestions for Study and Bibliographic Data*, 2nd edn (Philadelphia: W.B. Saunders and Company, 1917), p. 692.

118 'Medical Society of Victoria', p. 221.

119 Royal Society For the Prevention of Cruelty to Animals, *Vivisection. Royal Society For the Prevention of Cruelty to Animals and the Royal Commission*, 2nd edn (London: Smith, Elder, & Co., 1876), pp. xlii–xliv.

120 Edward Cardwell *et al.*, *Report of the Royal Commission on the Practice of Subjecting Live Animals to Experiments for Scientific Purposes; with Minutes of Evidence and Appendix*, vol. C.1397 and C.1397-I (London: Her Majesty's Stationery Office, 1876), p. 58.

CHAPTER FIVE

Legislators and other animals: foregrounding vivisection, 1876–95

On Christmas Eve, 1881, the Colony of Victoria passed an unlikely piece of legislation. Championed by a future Australian Prime Minister and vigorously supported by the colony's Premier and Attorney-General, *An Act for the Protection of Animals* codified Victoria as only the second legislature worldwide to formally regulate vivisection. Although patently derived from the United Kingdom's *Cruelty to Animals Act* of 1876, the antipodean debates and restrictions differed notably from this British precedent. Laying bare the operations of the colonial animal matrix, the Victorian Act codified experimental creatures alongside vermin, with predictable moral consequences. Indeed, the legislators drafting this bill were more concerned with defining suitable experimenters than protecting their animal subjects.

Both in its milieu and throughout the subsequent historiography, this colonial circumstance has largely eluded scrutiny. One reason is the enduring presumption that little animal experimentation occurred outside of Europe in the nineteenth century. Another is the low profile of animal protection movements in the Australian colonies. Why, then, would such arcane sentiments pass into Victoria's statute book?

Focusing on the 1880s, this chapter traces two discrete but germane colonial developments which legitimated vivisection in the authoritative generation of medical knowledge. The first is the passage of Victoria's *Protection of Animals Act* in the context of the animal welfare movements arising in late nineteenth-century Australia. The second is the ascent to global prominence of a novel remedy championed by a rural Victorian doctor who fervently – if sometimes hypocritically – denied the utility and veracity of animal experimentation. Encompassing both human and animal patients, snakebite antidotes provided the exemplar which united both of these colonial circumstances.

Vivisection, protection and nativism

Over 1870–1900, two discrete strands of animal protection evolved in colonial Australia, both intertwined with utilitarian evaluations of relative worth. The first was essentially conservative, encouraging the ongoing existence of favoured animal species. The second was predominantly moral, primarily a Benthamite concern to minimise suffering in individual creatures.[1] Within liberal legislatures, contends Siobhan O'Sullivan, 'there is a link between an animal's level of visibility and the extent to which that animal is well protected'.[2] Yet while her analysis focuses on economically equivalent animals such as horses, she overlooks beasts that are highly visible but of low – or negative – social and economic value.

Historically, such creatures constituted 'vermin'. Both the semantic and exegetic implications of this term were significant. Etymologically derived from worms, by the early modern era, 'vermin' encompassed not just serpents and sinuous quadrupeds like polecats, but numerous birds, bats, fish and insects.[3] Rather than a formal taxonomic order, by 1800 this pejorative defined a promiscuously anthropocentric schema of noxiousness suffusing British lay, legal and natural history discourses.[4] The moral justification for destroying vermin to protect laudable beasts – especially those aiding agricultural productivity – aligned blatantly economic motives with the injunction in Genesis 1:28 to exert 'dominion over the fish of the sea, and over the fowl of the air, and over every living thing that moveth upon the earth'.[5] As Thomas Dunlap's comparative ecological history of settler societies demonstrates, industrialised production of firearms, poisons and traps facilitated the wholesale extirpation of economically damaging and socially disruptive beasts, from hawks to unlicensed dogs.[6]

Undeniably visible, snakes vied only with rabbits as the most reviled creatures in late Victorian Australia. As its colonies transitioned to nationhood, argues sociologist Adrian Franklin, locally born nativists denigrated imported animals like rabbits as 'alien', concurrently elevating innocuous indigenes such as the kangaroo, emu and koala.[7] Amongst the earliest autochthonous birds to gain limited legislative protection was the kookaburra, which over 1850–1900 ascended from a despised chicken-killer to a lauded snake-destroyer (Figure 21).[8] Neither cultural visibility nor economic utility remained static characteristics within the colonial animal matrix.

Except, perhaps, for serpents. 'The snake was a metaphor for the dangers that lurked in the Australian bush', suggest Kevin Markwell and Nancy Cushing. Narratives which constructed venomous species 'as an object of scientific and natural history interest, as a risk to

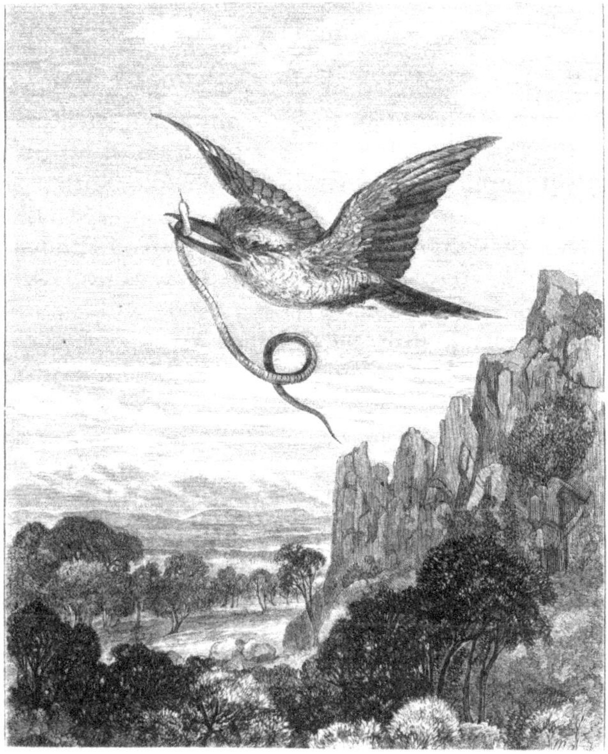

21 'The snake destroyer, the laughing jackass', *Illustrated Australian News*, 27 December 1876.

human safety, [and] as the object of a quest', they argue, 'are emblematic of modernist underpinnings of human–animal relations'.[9] An obsession with mastering such threatening beasts both valorised the Imperial hunting genre and predicated the extermination of creatures deemed dangerous to (neo-)colonial projects, from 'man-eaters' to mosquitoes.[10] As Australian settler Ada Cambridge recalled in 1903, 'in the bush it has ever been a point of honour ... to kill every snake you see, if possible, no matter how difficult the job, nor how great your impatience to be after other jobs'.[11]

Just as they did not profit from shifting statutory definitions of 'vermin', neither did snakes benefit when colonial parliamentarians turned to protecting beasts from cruelty. While laws constraining the suffering inflicted upon individual creatures developed largely from British precedents, colonial animal protection acts were necessitated by the uncertain reach of Imperial legislation. The first such law was enacted by John Franklin, Governor of Van Diemen's Land, in 1837. While his *Act for the Prevention of Cruelty to Animals* prospered, it paralleled a private bounty sanctioned by his wife Jane to rid the island of serpents. Otherwise, she was informed, snakes 'would rise up again in increased numbers on any cessation of hostilities, unless pursued to extermination'.[12] Although sporadic British attempts to slaughter Indian snakes often incensed locals – especially as cobras or *nāgas* represented divine serpent-lords for many Hindus, Buddhists and Jainists – antipodean serpents garnered few allies.[13] With convicts and colonists claiming £600 in bounties, Franklin's scheme soon foundered amidst social disorder and personal ridicule.

Over 1861–65, most Australian colonies adopted animal welfare clauses within their respective Police Acts to establish basic duties of care. Societies promoting animal welfare subsequently emerged in Victoria (1871), New South Wales (1873), South Australia (1875), Tasmania (1878), Queensland (1876, but effectively 1883) and Western Australia (1892). Their educational and moralising missions were bolstered by legislative agitation and recognition of their inspectors as pseudo-constables under relevant laws.[14] But as in contemporary Europe, welfare crusades were directed almost exclusively towards pets and urban working animals; farm fauna and wild beasts rarely warranted consideration. In settler settings, as Daniel Gilfoyle has detailed in his study of *fin de siècle* veterinary immunology in Southern Africa, animal welfare qualms were less likely to inhibit the investigation or adoption of vaccines designed specifically for livestock.[15] Moreover, the absence of organised antivivisection agitation in the Cape Colony enabled the use of 'vermin' – rabbits – in developing a rabies vaccine to protect humans and their domestic creatures.[16]

If the colonial remit of British legislation remained unclear, laws against cruel experiments found few champions in Australia – especially for snakebite investigations. Notwithstanding an 1883 pamphlet enjoining Victorian children to avoid 'acting towards animals as if they were mere bodies of skin, bone, and flesh without feelings, hopes, fears, or wants like ourselves', colonial publics enjoyed spectacles pitting snakes against domesticated animals into the 1890s (Figure 22).[17]

Throughout the nineteenth century, the United Kingdom provided the emotional heart for Anglophone antivivisection agitation. Receiving Queen Victoria's assent in 1840, the Royal Society for the Prevention of Cruelty to Animals remained both the most politically potent and globally influential of British animal welfare bodies. However, by the 1870s its social conservatism – particularly

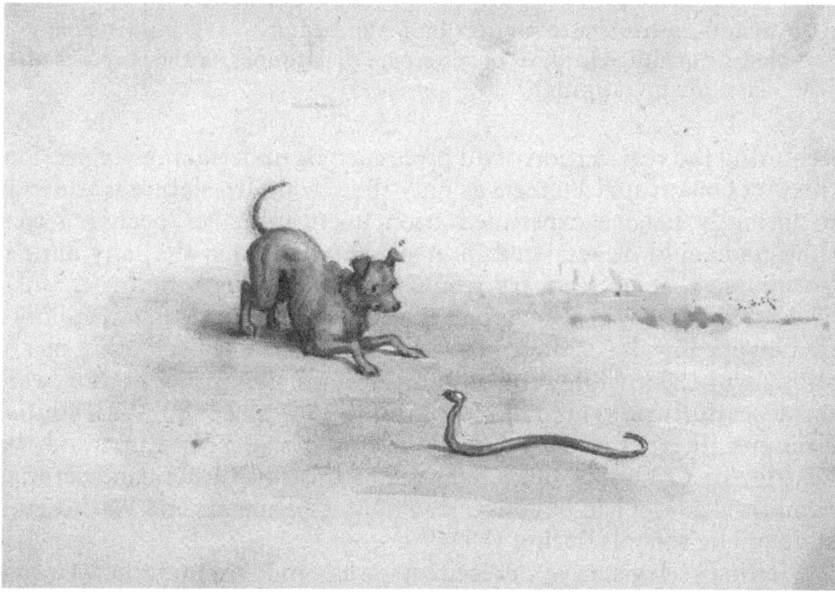

22 George Goodwin Kilburne, 'Study of a dog attacking a snake', *c.*1883.

an unwillingness to veto animal experimentation – inspired numerous offshoot groups. Indeed by 1883, over a quarter of the 506 animal protection societies identified by a global survey were determinedly antivivisectionist.[18] In that year the first American Anti-Vivisection Society was founded in Philadelphia, geographically and temporally flourishing alongside the continent's expanding medical research culture.[19] Such campaigns, suggests Anita Guerrini, were as Arcadian as they were abolitionist: 'animals represented a connection with nature and a rural past that was rapidly disappearing, while science foreshadowed a modern world of ceaseless change and instability'.[20]

Animal welfare rarely troubled Australian participants in snakebite demonstrations. This ethical apathy renders all the more remarkable legislation passed by the Victorian Parliament on 24 December 1881. Defining cruelty as 'the intentional infliction upon any animal of pain that in its kind or its degree or its object or its circumstances is unreasonable', *An Act for the Protection of Animals* exempted from prosecution suffering perpetrated:

(*a*) In the extermination of rabbits foxes wild dogs or vermin; or
(*b*) In the hunting snaring trapping shooting or taking of any animal not in a domestic state; or

(*c*) In any experiment or vivisection performed upon any animal by any legally qualified medical or veterinary practitioner for the purposes of scientific investigation.[21]

Requiring the registration of all professionals undertaking vivisection, this Act constituted Victoria as only the second legislature worldwide to formally licence experimentation upon animals. Specifying that subjects should be rendered insensible to pain, and that any animal 'so injured that its recovery would involve serious suffering ... shall be destroyed', it was also among the earliest to provide any regulatory framework for vivisecting.[22] Bavaria had constrained scientific use of animals in 1833, while bills prohibiting animal experimentation were unsuccessfully presented in New York in 1867 and 1880. With similar attempts likewise defeated in Massachusetts, Pennsylvania and the District of Columbia over 1893–1906, the sole American victories comprised a brief ban of vivisection in Massachusetts and Washington state public schools during 1894–95.[23]

Victoria's legislative precedent was indubitably the United Kingdom's *Cruelty to Animals Act* 1876. Although Britain's shift towards animal experimentation was gradual, proposes Richard French, 'if a single year be chosen as a turning point, that year must be 1870'.[24] Aware of precedents dating from the 1830s, in 1871 a British Association for the Advancement of Science committee of anatomists and physiologists proposed a code to govern animal experiments.[25] Its emphasis on suitably skilled operators, well-equipped laboratories and almost mandatory anaesthesia did not allay rising public opprobrium. A Royal Commission on the Practice of Subjecting Live Animals to Experiments for Scientific Purposes, tabled on 8 January 1876, asserted that vivisection offered justifiable – if sometimes unforeseeable – benefits both for medical and veterinary pedagogy, and in furthering the prevention and treatment of disease.[26]

Key to the resultant *Cruelty to Animals Act* was the biological remit of juridical protection. Each person experimenting upon vertebrates required a Home Office licence, alongside special certificates to vivisect cats, dogs, horses, mules or asses.[27] Importantly, the Act's purlieu encompassed frogs, a common experimental subject valued equally for its moral invisibility and epistemological status as a generic quadruped.[28] Although antivivisection agitation escalated over the following decades, from August 1876 the Act provided both legislative approbation and legal parameters for British experimentalists.[29] Moreover, in August 1881 the International Medical Congress in London promulgated a conspicuous endorsement of vivisection, asserting the autonomy of professional science and medicine from their former deference to aristocratic, ecclesiastic and judicial fetters.[30] By 1884, amid escalating numbers of vivisectors and procedures, the Home Office devolved its adjudicatory role to the pro-experimentation Association for the Advancement of Medicine by Research. Thus Britain provided a global template not for abolishing vivisection, but for its promulgation within a largely self-regulatory framework.[31]

In contrast to the public outcry in Britain, Victoria's 1881 legislation was short on sentiment. Indeed, its terms directly equated experimental animals with vermin and 'useless' wild beasts. Yet its impetus likely originated with the Victorian Society for the Prevention of Cruelty to Animals (VSPCA), the earliest such antipodean organisation when founded in 1871. It took a profoundly pragmatic attitude towards animal welfare, an 1880 pamphlet declaring that animals embodied 'an inferior, not a different, organisation to our own', thus purveying a fundamental acceptance of the biological homologies and ethical hierarchies underpinning vivisection.[32]

Unsurprisingly, experimental animals were absent from the bill first presented to the Victorian Legislative Assembly on 5 October 1881. Its architect was prominent VSPCA member, nativist and vegetarian, Alfred Deakin, later Australia's second prime minister. Upon its first reading, however, pharmacist-politician Joseph Bosisto proposed 'saving words for the protection of persons conducting experiments with a view to the prevention or cure of disease'.[33] His focus was explicitly the practitioner, not the subject. The colony's Premier and Attorney-General, Bryan O'Loghlen, then mooted a clause to exempt animal experiments from prosecutions for cruelty, rejecting the wholesale adoption of British regulations which might allow sentimental busybodies to constrain legitimate medical inquiry. His fellow parliamentarians demurred when obstetrician Louis Smith proposed that 'it would be well if the contemplated immunity was extended to University professors'; in 1881 the colony's sole medical professor was George Halford.[34]

Where parliamentary debate encompassed experimental animals, snakes were doubly prominent. If serpents themselves were expendable, studying their poison overrode consideration for envenomed experimental animals – as the British Royal Commission had asserted in 1875. 'How could the action of snake poison … be investigated, or the remedial action of galvanism have been discovered, without cruelty to dogs?' queried Smith, recalling his own snakebite 'studies' on stage in the 1860s. Likewise, a clause specifying mandatory anaesthesia was diluted to require merely analgesia because, as pastoralist James Buchanan elaborated in the Legislative Council, 'this provision would render experiments on snakes, for the purpose of discovering an antidote to snake poison, altogether useless'.[35] Snakebite was thus foregrounded in the Victorian Parliament's otherwise brief exchanges over animal experimentation. Indeed, in contrast with Britain, *An Act for the Protection of Animals* passed quite painlessly.

A dead letter? Victoria's vivisection legislation in practice

On 3 September 1883, George Halford became the first practitioner beyond Britain granted a Vivisection Licence, distinguishing him as a *professional* physiologist. Its conditions were determined both by the 1881 Act and supplementary regulations directed by the Governor in Council. Despite jurist Philip Jamieson's claim that Victoria's Act broke with British precedent because it did not specify licensing requirements, these gubernatorial regulations clearly derived from the UK's *Cruelty to Animals Act*.[36] Yet, unlike the exhaustive pages of British restrictions, Victorian provisos appeared both more succinct and far less permissive of exemptions.

It is noteworthy that the Chief Secretary's Office compiled Victorian Vivisection Licences within the same record book as Licences to Practice Anatomy and permits to hold public entertainments.[37] There were certainly grounds for confusion. In October 1883, barely a month after Halford gained his Victorian licence, a scandal threatened in New South Wales. Sydney University's new Professor of Physiology and Anatomy – Thomas Anderson Stuart – was caught with a dog in his dissecting room. His adamant denials that this 'stray' was intended for vivisection laid clear Stuart's presumption that colonial animal experimentation was bound in principle by British law. Thomas Belgrave, the colony's recently appointed Anatomy Inspector, was similarly uncertain.[38] Ultimately, no prosecution ensued, and the New South Wales Parliament did not address animal welfare aspects of vivisection until 1928. Edward Stirling, physiology lecturer at the continent's third medical school in Adelaide, had been refused a British Vivisection Licence in 1880. Later prominent in South Australia's Royal Society for the Prevention of Cruelty to Animals, his investigations favoured morbid anatomy and palaeontology over vivisection.

The Victorian conjunction of permits and licences questioned not only where vivisection could legally be performed, but to what ends. 'Any exhibition to the general public', ran the UK Act, 'whether admitted on payment of money or gratuitously, of experiments on living animals calculated to give pain shall be illegal.'[39] Victoria's Act contained no equivalent clause; neither its intent nor letter constrained public demonstration of snakebite antidotes. Until Federation, such shows remained frequent and prominent, oftentimes dignified by medical or scientific figures. That envenomed animals became distressed was often painfully apparent. That their suffering was left untended – at least in creatures not receiving the 'antidote' – was integral to the display.

Halford's Vivisection Licence, moreover, proved a dead letter. Apparently ceasing physiological investigations after 1877, it says much of the limited awareness of the Victorian Act that he was not among the 468 practitioners listed in the global *Vivisectors' Directory*, compiled in 1884 by two prominent antivivisection societies. His contemporaries certainly featured. Alongside Silas Weir Mitchell – America's champion of physiological experiment – Britons whose animal studies explored snake venoms and antidotes included George Harley, Joseph Fayrer, Vincent Richards and Thomas Lauder Brunton. Others vivisecting with venoms included Brazilian physiologist João Batista Lacerda, French doctor (Émile Julien) Armand Gautier, Russian neuropathologist Vladimir Roth and Japanese physiologist Kenji Osawa.[40] Moreover, by the 1880s barely a handful of British doctors decried vivisection.[41] Yet in Victoria it was only in 1888 that a second Vivisection Licence was granted – to Halford's new physiology demonstrator, James Barrett, already awarded a British licence. Victoria's third licensee, surgeon Stephen Caffyn, waited until 1890.[42]

Animal experiments continued regardless and were never confined to 'legally qualified medical or veterinary practitioners'. Among the most startling was presented by plant pathologist Daniel McAlpine to the Royal Society of Victoria in June 1890. Killing copperhead snakes via decapitation or chloroform, McAlpine measured how soon their hearts stopped beating and the distance each excised organ travelled along a moistened plate.[43] Tabulating results gained from similar experiments in fish, frogs, tortoises, chickens, rabbits and kittens, nobody in McAlpine's esteemed audience queried whether he possessed a Vivisection Licence. He didn't.

Accountability was similarly slipshod. Prompted by the VSPCA, Governor George Phipps requested quarterly reports of Halford's animal experiments. Commencing 30 September 1883, they were to detail the following:

(a) The kind of animal used
(b) The purpose of the experiment
(c) What fresh knowledge, if any, has been obtained by the experiment
(d) The anæsthetic administered, and what dose was used
(e) The period elapsing between the drugging of the animal and its restoration to consciousness, or its destruction
(f) Whence the animal was obtained, and how it was disposed of afterwards.[44]

Halford did no such thing. He provided just one return, in March 1884, thereafter intermittently informing the Colonial Secretary's office that 'he had not had recourse to vivisection'.[45] Likely with his consent, Halford's Vivisection Licence was revoked on 20 March 1888, the void in physiological demonstrations presumably being filled by Barrett. Yet in 1894, and again in 1897, Halford admitted to conducting venom and antidote experiments in dogs and rabbits. He was even encouraged by the recently appointed Chief Justice of Victoria, John Madden, who wrote on his judicial letterhead extolling the Professor's 'fires of energetic investigation'.[46]

Vivisection was therefore neither unusual, nor controversial, in the one jurisdiction outside of Britain which formally regulated the practice before 1900. In contrast to the escalating agitation in Britain after 1876, few animal welfare groups attempted to limit experimentation anywhere in Australia until the British Union for the Abolition of Vivisection established branches in Melbourne (1924) and Sydney (1928).[47] Nevertheless, vivisection clauses comparable to Victoria's were gradually incorporated into prevention of cruelty legislation in Queensland (1901), South Australia (1908), Western Australia (1912), Tasmania (1925) and New South Wales (1928).[48]

Colonial animal protection organisations were more concerned with the abuse of animals as a brutalising influence on proletarians than in preserving creatures for their inherent value. Such sensibilities troubled few colonists, and even fewer doctors. If experimental physiology remained uncommon in the colonial antipodes, the quest to remedy snakebite proved a vital exception. Snakes were no ordinary vermin; they were extraordinarily visible. Furthermore, snakebite studies degraded the moral standing of their fellow animal participants, denying mandatory anaesthesia for these 'insensible' experimental instruments. This devaluation accelerated when a putative remedy reinvigorated colonial venom investigations as the nineteenth century closed.

Snakes, strychnine and suicide

With snakebite reports spread thin across the colonies, Australian venom science remained quiescent throughout the 1880s. Indeed, it was a severe redback spider bite in 1882 which prompted a Victorian general practitioner to experiment with subcutaneously injecting strychnine into a two-year-old boy. When his young patient recovered, Augustus Mueller was seduced by the 'almost magical action' of his remedy and soon extended it to snakebite.[49]

This Prussian immigrant had settled in rural Yackandandah in 1863, gaining equal respect as a doctor and vigneron (Figure 23). By February

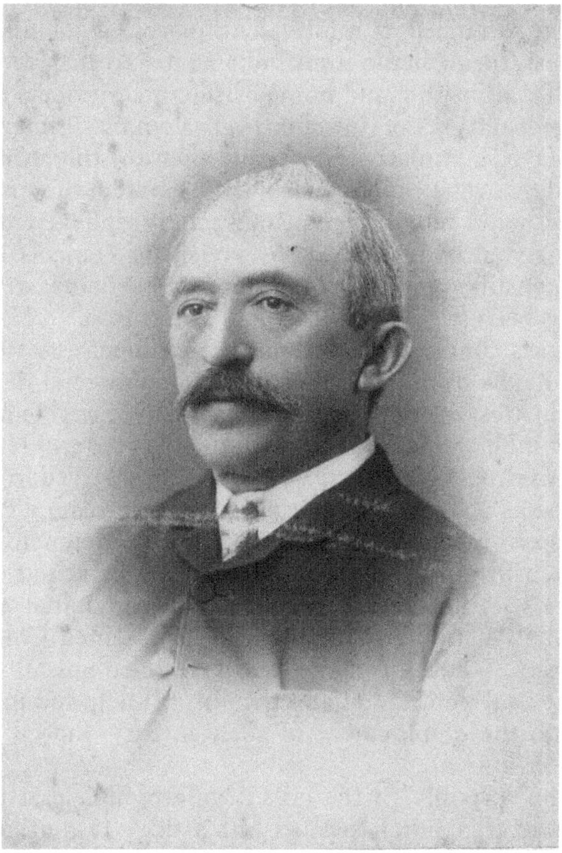

23 Studio portrait of Augustus Mueller, *c.*1880s.

1888 he felt impelled to register his discovery with Victoria's Central Board of Health, but before a reward might be considered – advised the colony's Chief Medical Officer – Mueller 'would have to demonstrate the efficacy of [his] antidote on lower animals, and also bring the matter before the Medical Society of Victoria'.[50] Eschewing vivisection, Mueller addressed the Society on 2 May 1888, couching his plan as a complete scientific theory derived from three decades of observing snakebitten patients and domestic animals. When Melbourne's elite practitioners summarily dismissed this spartan clinical evidence, Mueller turned to Sydneysider John Mildred Creed, editor of the *Australasian Medical Gazette*. Creed immediately championed Mueller's campaign, in 1890 urging 'the whole of the Australian Governments to ... publish the facts as stated, for the information of the people'.[51]

Strychnine occupied a multivalent place in colonial Australia. Entering western medicine from India as a sixteenth-century plague cure, by 1888 allopathic and homeopathic practitioners alike widely employed preparations of *Strychnos nux vomica*. Primarily a stimulant, it displayed cumulative effects and a narrow therapeutic window. Too high a dose overstimulated the nervous system to cause twitching, then spasms, before tetanic convulsions fatally asphyxiated the patient. Unsurprisingly, although praised by vivisector François Magendie in his widely consulted formulary of scientific medicine, strychnine had for centuries been stigmatised as a dramatic poison.[52]

Strychnine's course through the nineteenth-century world charted a dynamic nexus of imperial, industrial, commercial, legal and vernacular identities, many predicated on equally unstable renderings of 'science'. In India, remarks David Arnold, the resort of Hindu doctors to 'dangerous drugs' such as *nux vomica* seeds 'served in the rhetoric of the period as a significant site of contestation and differentiation' against western medicine.[53] Beyond British developments in toxicology and forensics – foregrounded by several spectacular mid-century murder trials – strychnine poisoning of Aboriginal people 'like foxes' on the Australian contract frontier alarmed Colonial Office administrators.[54] But for many antipodean colonists, a profusion of home medical guides and an ethos of self-help fed into a culture conducive to the employment of such active – indeed, spectacular – remedies.[55]

Strychnine certainly fit the bill. Regularly broadcast to eliminate 'vermin' and often purchased 'to kill a dog', it routinely featured in suicide reports, leading antipodean pharmacists to campaign for uniform poisons regulation. Regardless, reported the *Chemist and Druggist of Australasia*, over 1887–1900 strychnine advanced from a minor constituent of dispensed medicines to their commonest ingredient.[56]

Yet doctors were initially sceptical when, in January 1889, Mueller presented his snakebite antidote to the Second Intercolonial Medical Congress of Australasia in Melbourne. Remarkably, despite prompting robust discussion, his session was omitted from the Congress proceedings.[57] To Mueller there was no mystery: it had been 'deliberately suppressed and left out' by the organisers, a coterie of senior Medical Society of Victoria members.[58] Creed responded by running the article in his *Gazette* and securing Mueller a prominent place at the third Congress in 1892. Ironically, this conference series had been instigated precisely to draw the profession together. First held in Adelaide in 1887, it trumped the Australasian Association for the Advancement of Science by a year. Such was the quest to make antipodean medicine scientific that organisers hoped – vainly as it turned out – to align these two intercolonial symposia.[59]

But 'science' carried vastly different connotations for Australia's diverse practitioners. To Mueller, it comprised a comprehensive theory bolstered by clinical success. Thus he invoked British doctors versed in Indian venoms to propound his 'law of reduced motor nerve force emanating from the motor nerve centres'.[60] Snake venoms, Mueller argued, primarily attacked the motor nerve ends, not the blood. Poison crept through the body, paralysing skeletal muscles, the heart, lungs and especially the fine neuromotor control of capillary dilation. The resultant diapedesis disseminated blood into the abdominal cavity and kidneys, accounting for the characteristic faintness and weak pulse. The 'purely physiological' action of strychnine was therefore 'exactly the reverse of that of snake-poison', restoring muscular tone 'with the unerring certainty and precision of a chemical test'.[61]

Despite asserting the general applicability of his law, Mueller blamed idiosyncratic manifestations of envenomation upon interspecies variations. Such disparities, Mueller attested, obviated vivisectional data. 'It is not by experiments on animals', he entreated the Intercolonial Medical Congress in 1892, 'but by a hearty co-operation of all Australian medical men, that this subject will receive the elucidation so urgently called for.'[62]

Mueller's objections were both humane and pragmatic. He consistently professed his 'perfect horror of vivisection, of torturing poor animals for the sake of experiments, which ... have been conspicuously barren of results'.[63] Lacking a Vivisection Licence, this Victorian doctor nevertheless killed snakes to extract their poison glands, mixing venom with a chicken's blood before injecting it into another hen. Eschewing anaesthetic, he exposed snail and frog hearts to record the paralysing effects of tiger snake venom. Proudly rural, he cited snakebites in domesticates ranging from cats to bullocks as evidence of venom potency – and to vindicate his remedy. Moreover, Mueller's intellectual touchstone was an obscure – at least in Australia – doctoral dissertation published in German by Russian investigator Aleksandr Feoktistow. Having injected viper and rattlesnake venoms into 400 creatures spanning the animal kingdom, Feoktistow's experiments in higher vertebrates were cited by Mueller – without irony – as homologues for human envenomation.[64]

While Sharon Wallace asserts that Mueller was misguided in opposing vivisection because 'his peers expected no less', the volume of clinical material proffered in his support suggests otherwise.[65] He was not posing as a clinical savant; in John Pickstone's terminology, Mueller's modus was museological-diagnostic, building predictive structures from collected observations. Sharing ambivalence toward the heuristic and moral value of vivisection, Mueller perpetuated Halford's exploratory approach to scientific discovery. What neither represented was experimental science, 'the controlled production of new phenomena in laboratories'.[66] This emphasis on command and production, Pickstone argues, established a hierarchy between the creation and mastery of knowledge – what Ohad Parnes has termed 'epistemological sovereignty' – and its application in quotidian clinical practice.[67]

Déjà vu: Halford, Mueller and injected remedies

As a snakebite antidote, strychnine was hardly new. Employed as early as 1861, by 1868 its hypodermic injection was proposed both in Australia and by Joseph Fayrer and Vincent Richards in India.[68] If Mueller, like many colleagues, had abandoned Halford's ammonia injection by the late 1870s, numerous contemporaries drew the obvious parallels between their techniques. Indeed, Mueller remarked wryly in 1889, cures effected by his treatment were sometimes attributed to Halford's practice.[69] Occasionally, clinicians employed both injections.

While 1876 had effectively halted antipodean venom research, it also heralded a new reductivist approach in Indian, American and European studies. Now seen as complex chemical mixtures, 'venoms' were no longer singular. But there remained no teleological certainty that Australian snake venoms would be similarly fractionated. In Brazil, from 1878 João Baptista Lacerda undertook vivisections to generate an antidote against snake venoms. Convinced that the toxic principle was a single substance that could be chemically neutralised by subcutaneous or intravenous injections of permanganate of potash solution, his experiments culminated in dramatically reviving a snakebitten dog before Emperor Pedro II in 1881. Within a month, Lacerda's remedy was being injected by physicians, surgeons, pharmacists and laity, generating demand for a German-made kit comprising a syringe and his chemical preparation. Escalating local adoption soon saw Lacerda invoking 'clinical facts' to counter theoretical and experimental challenges from French and British vivisectors, including Fayrer, Richards and Brunton. If the absence of a detailed scientific explanation mitigated against European acceptance of Lacerda's claims, suggests Ana Vimieiro Gomes, recourse to his antidote remained widespread across the Americas into the 1940s.[70]

In Australia, Mueller's strychnine injection likewise promised clinical unity amidst looming diversity and complexity. 'The simplicity of the working of your antidote', wrote one rural practitioner in 1894, 'is such that after demonstrating it once to a room-full of people, each one expressed himself confident of administering it.'[71] One corollary of Mueller's theorem was that no single dose was uniformly effective: neutralising venom required repeated injections until muscular spasms appeared. This phenomenon also proved diagnostically useful: if strychnine injection produced no twitches, the patient truly had been envenomed. Although he considered alcohol useless for snakebite, Mueller agreed with many that venom completely eliminated its intoxicating effects. Thus, the onset of inebriation after challenge with spirits indicated when strychnine had vanquished the venom. All eminently practical.

As cases multiplied, Mueller's certitude divided the Australian medical community. Garnering uneven support from British and colonial periodicals in medicine and pharmacy, by 1892 even the antagonistic *Australian Medical Journal* felt impelled to publish cases. Across 1890–96, the *Australasian Medical Gazette* ran over 100 cases of strychnine injection for snakebite from doctors, pharmacists, laity and the constabulary. After petitioning by Creed, the New South Wales Inspector-General of Police issued a colony-wide circular on 2 March 1891 requiring his men to collate reports of snakebite 'to arrive at right conclusions as to the efficacy of the use of strychnine by hypodermic injections in cases of snake-bite, which it is asserted authoritatively has been to the present almost unfailing in apparently desperate cases'.[72]

This formal approbation eased the transition of strychnine injection from last resort to first preference. Venom expert Charles Campbell suggests that many reported snakebites were likely not life-threatening – at least, not until strychnine was superadded.[73] In privileging clinical testimony over vivisectional testing, the medical debate replayed Halford's saga of the 1870s, although the Medical Society of Victoria refused to conduct animal experiments to evaluate strychnine injection. Indeed, amongst practitioners it was dosing, not animal testing, which proved most contentious. As failures mounted – especially amongst children – doctors declined to pump unprecedented levels of this poison into their patients. 'Better not use the antidote at all than use it timidly', Mueller countered.[74]

The injection apparatus itself was a critical actant. In 1868, Halford's approach had coincided with accelerating availability of hypodermic syringes. By 1890 this technology was thoroughly regularised. Mueller did not overstate his remedy's popularity by claiming in 1893 that there was 'scarcely a settlement in the Australian bush now where it is not kept in pocket-cases containing [a] hypodermic syringe and printed directions for use' (Figure 24).[75] Extending Iwan Morus's convincing argument that Victorian audiences for scientific

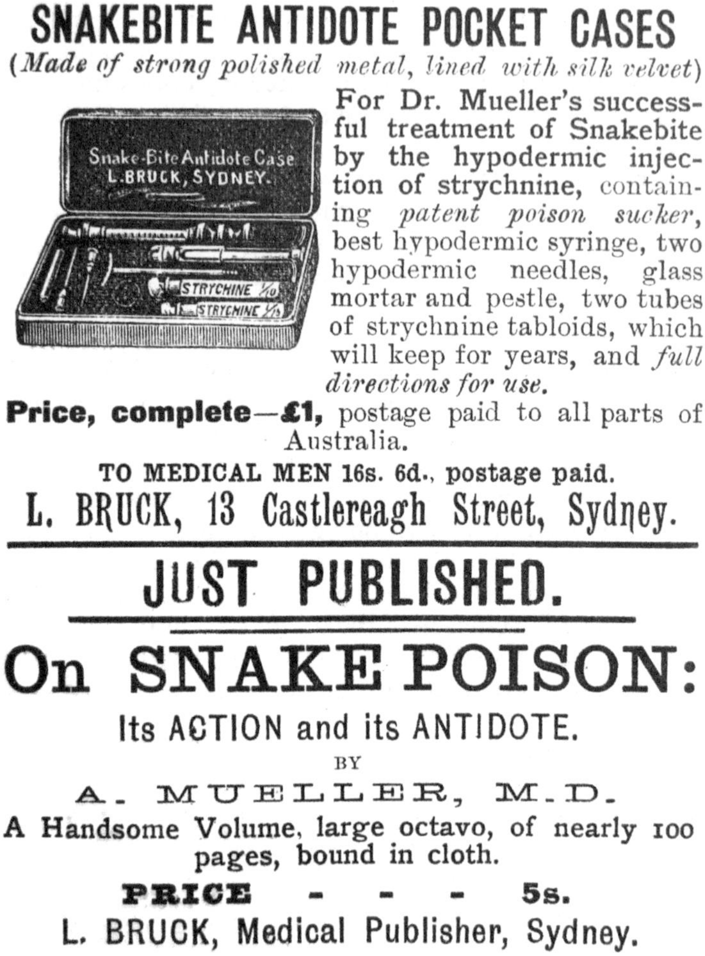

24 Advertisement for snakebite antidote pocket cases, *Australasian Medical Gazette,* March 1893.

spectacles 'constituted themselves as the public through their active participation in performances', colonists purchasing a snakebite kit crafted their own parochial assemblages of apparatus, enactment and observation to affirm that strychnine truly constituted 'scientific medicine'.[76]

Not only were syringes ever-present; by 1890 the emerging pharmaceutical houses – especially the British Burroughs–Wellcome and American Parke, Davis & Co. – had introduced tabloids to standardise dosing of hypodermically injected drugs. Local firms such as Felton,

Grimwade & Co. followed suit, as did Brisbane surgeon and apothecary Richard Rendle. His strychnine injection kit contained a popular booklet on both venomous serpents and snakebite treatment, furthermore warning of the dangerous variability between competing strychnine presentations.[77] In January 1892 the *Chemist and Druggist of Australasia* summarised strychnine doses for snakebite cases. 'Every chemist in snake districts should commit these directions to memory', the journal warned, 'and should have always at hand all the necessary materials'.[78]

With snakebite kits proliferating, Yackandandah chemist Matthew Rome proved more entrepreneurial than Mueller. By mid-1889 he was marketing a neat case containing a syringe, hypodermic needles, a vial of strychnine and Mueller's instructions. In 1891 Rome patented a refined solution 'for application of a remedial antidote in cases of snakebite, & c., without the aid of a doctor'.[79] Mueller himself praised his many lay converts who were 'even more successful because less timid than many medical men'.[80] Matching the cost of Halford's and Julius Berncastle's 1860s snakebite kits – a guinea – by 1894 Rome's case competed with a rival chloride of lime injection. Despite favourable reports from Halford, however, the latter antidote proved evanescent.

The ubiquity of hypodermic syringes was symptomatic of a wider transformation in clinical medicine. As Stanley Reiser has argued, over 1870–90 a widespread introduction of diagnostic devices 'drew the physician into a universe of physical changes concealed from the natural senses'.[81] From microscopes to sphygmomanometers, these technologies also included physico-chemical processes and bacteriological cultures for analysing gastric contents, urine, blood and serum. From the fever chart to the radiograph, the transcription of such results hallmarked modern medicine.[82] After 1895, such apparatuses transmogrified venom science. In the interim, Mueller's nemesis comprised a different form of quantification: statistics.

Mueller's challengers: statistics and the subcontinent

If subcutaneous strychnine approached medical orthodoxy across Australia by 1892, the following year proved Mueller's *annus mirabilis*. Reviewing his 1893 monograph – *On Snake Poison, its Action and its Antidote* – the *Chemist and Druggist of Australasia* asserted that 'the case is almost proved'.[83] In his April 1893 presidential address to the New South Wales Branch of the British Medical Association, Creed lauded the adoption of Mueller's treatment throughout the Australian colonies and its official endorsement in India.[84] Yet the ageing Mueller declined to take his prime place at the Third Intercolonial Medical

Congress of Australasia in September 1892. Instead its director, Sydney Hospital physician (Louis) Ralston Huxtable, robustly critiqued Mueller's swelling support base.

Counterbalancing what he portrayed as an impressionistic parade of clinical miracles, Huxtable collected data. Over 1891–92 he induced the local Board of Health to circularise New South Wales practitioners, seeking the number of snakebites attended, modes of treatment used and outcomes. Forwarding similar questionnaires to Victorian and Queensland country doctors, Huxtable also requested itemised returns of snakebite deaths over 1881–91 from statistical departments across the mainland. He furthermore tabulated all snakebite cases printed in the *Australasian Medical Gazette* since Mueller's announcement of 1888.[85] Collating nearly 500 reports, Huxtable provided the most comprehensive snapshot of snakebite in colonial Australia.[86] His primary conclusion was that 'in the great majority of cases strong and healthy adults recover from the bite of even our most venomous Australian species without the aid of treatment'; children were another matter. Damning alcohol and forced exercise, he blamed contemporary treatments for hastening death, associating strychnine with 13.2% mortality against 4.1% without.[87]

Two months later, Melbourne University's Demonstrator in Physiology, James Barrett, presented similar data to the Royal Society of Victoria. Via returns from the colony's statist, he concluded that snakes had despatched only 125 Australians over 1881–90. Killing one citizen per 17,886 and accounting for 0.5% of violent ends, snakebite represented 'one of the most insignificant causes of death in our midst'. Regarding experimentation, Barrett – still unique in possessing both British and Victorian Vivisection Licences – was dogmatic. 'There is only one method by which the value of strychnia as a remedy may be settled, viz., by resort to experiments on animals on which the action of snake poison does not to all appearances differ materially from that in the case of man.'[88] This assertion was endorsed by his eminent audience, including herpetologist Charles Frost, Government Astronomer Robert Ellery, and the Professors of Biology from Melbourne and Sydney Universities – Walter Baldwin Spencer and William Haswell.

Ignoring Barrett, Mueller dismissed Huxtable's data as the folly of townsfolk who underrated both Australian snakes and the first-aid taught to every schoolchild and known to every bushman.[89] His own allies were numerous, including the most revered scientific figure in *fin de siècle* Victoria: botanist and explorer, Baron Ferdinand von Mueller. Not directly related, the Muellers were familiar, probably through shared interests in viticulture and phylloxera. In 1888 the Baron forwarded his namesake's musings on strychnine to the respected German experimental medicine journal, *Virchows Archiv*.[90] Prompted by von Mueller, in 1894 'Dr. Macher, Yarkandandah, Victoria' also touted his injection to the well-established *Therapeutic Gazette*, detailing 'many authenticated cases to prove to your American countrymen the correctness of this important discovery, so that it will gain ground and benefit a distant country'.[91] It didn't, yet American practitioners were also urged to consider Mueller's data by Leonhard Stejneger, Curator of Reptiles and Batrachians at the Smithsonian Institution. While the diversity of snake venoms saw many 'antidotes' falter, Stejneger opined, the curative 'which really seems to come up to all reasonable expectation, is a poison scarcely less terrible than the snake venom itself, viz. *strychnine*'.[92]

America, however, was never the main string in Mueller's bow. Soon attracting interest in India, by 1890 news of a Raj prize for an effective snakebite remedy saw him targeting the Indian Government and the President of its Medical Board, Fayrer. In March 1892, Creed – now a Member of Parliament – secured the assistance of the New South Wales Governor to convey Mueller's kit and directions directly to the Viceroy of India, who passed them to his medical department.[93] That September, Mueller convinced the Governor of Victoria to forward details of his remedy to Britain's Secretary of State for the Colonies, George Robinson, who placed Mueller's epistle before Queen Victoria herself. Her Majesty instructed Robinson to request that the Indian Government 'give careful trials to Dr. Mueller's methods under the supervision of a complete medical committee at Calcutta, and also in selected hospitals'.[94] Initially setting a three-year probation, an 1894 interim analysis suggested a further two years of monitoring. Embracing his royal patronage, Mueller wrote directly to the Indian Government in December 1892 to ensure a fair trial. His first condition: 'Experiment on the lower animals be dispensed with as misleading.'[95]

Although Fayrer accorded Mueller more credence than he had Halford, it again appeared that the 1870s were being replayed. Indian clinicians initially doubted both the toxicity of Australian snakes and the veracity of Australian practitioners. Yet when Creed appealed for Indian cases in December 1891, a reply came from Ram Prasad Banerjee at the Northern India Salt Revenue Hospital in Rajasthan. Amid Banerjee's eight snakebite cases, what startled antipodean doctors was his administration of up to 4 grains (~ 260 g) of strychnine: the medicolegally accepted lethal dose was 0.5–2 grains.[96] When his taxonomy was also queried, Banerjee protested that 'one or two writers on Indian snakes and their experiments on dogs and cats' did not override local knowledge.[97] Nevertheless, Surgeon-Captain John Tull Walsh requested – and received – Banerjee's preserved snakes.

Correcting their identification at the Indian Museum, he suggested that readers accept only cases proffered by white medical officers; the *Australasian Medical Gazette* demurred.[98]

Indeed, as subcontinental accounts accumulated, Australian and Indian periodicals regularly reprinted each other's reports, leading the *Indian Medical Gazette* to propose extensive trials. When Joshua Duke – Surgeon-Lieutenant-Colonel in the Bengal Army – summarised 37 cases of strychnine injection for the First Indian Medical Congress in December 1894, he declared Mueller's method 'the best, in fact the only remedy to be relied on ... [when] carried out with the boldness recommended by him'.[99] Without dismissing vivisection, Duke proposed a more definitive test: inviting Mueller to India to inject six condemned criminals bitten by deadly serpents. The elderly Australian doctor declined.

But if Mueller had forestalled animal experiments, he could not forever hold off sceptics who invoked the 1873–74 Indian Snakebite Commission. By 1894, such calls reached a clamour, culminating in a paper delivered to the South Indian Branch of the British Medical Association by Robert Elliot, Professor of Biology at the Madras Medical College.[100] Testing strychnine against venoms from 'the most deadly snakes of Asia, Australia, America, and Africa, and especially the Indian cobra', Elliott recorded not a single recovery in 30 envenomed frogs, lizards, fowls, ducks, hares, guinea pigs, dogs, pigs, goats or monkeys.[101] From 1895, the verisimilitude of clinical case reports faded before the mantra of modern vivisectors such as Indian Medical Service stalwart David Cunningham, who asserted that 'it is only by means of accurate experiment that the actual value of any alleged antidote can be fairly estimated, for it is only by experiment that the actual lethal properties of any particular venom can be determined'.[102]

As the probationary period for strychnine injection expired in India, Mueller lamented the absence of official recognition for his services to Australia.[103] Dying in 1898, his remedy outlived him, slowly fading from international reference texts but sustaining local adherents. In 1914, the first Australian textbook of therapeutics commended Mueller's method '*if used boldly yet scientifically*'.[104] Indeed, a 1906 collation of Australian snakebite reports acknowledged its frequent clinical use, contradicting negative vivisectional data to suggest that case fatality was identical in snakebitten patients treated with or without strychnine (34.5% vs 35.0%).[105] This series, however, was the only one not to show that strychnine actively killed patients, with bans on its sale for snakebite commencing with Queensland in 1913. Its use nevertheless persisted into the 1920s, being recommended by Sydney's Royal Alexandria Hospital for Children as late as 1951.[106]

Medical accounts of the rise of subcutaneous strychnine for snake-bite render its demise both desirable and inevitable.[107] Yet in 1893 it embodied scientific medicine in the Australian colonies and, to a large extent, India. Its trajectory was paralleled by the euphoric ascent and disheartening decline of Robert Koch's proto-biomedical tuberculin therapy over the same moment, an evanescence as apparent in Australia as in Germany.[108] Much of strychnine's rapid acceptance and widespread adoption can be attributed to Mueller's cogent rationale and robust clinical guidelines, the regularisation of precisely dosed administration, and cumulative practitioner testimonials. Conversely, its slide from ubiquity was unspectacular, driven by a mounting death toll – especially in children – and a quiet disquiet over adverse statistical and experimental data.

If vivisection occupied an ambiguous place in late colonial medical heuristics, it was rarely critiqued on ethical grounds – except, erratically, by Mueller. Vivisection Licenses remained a rarity in *fin de siècle* Victoria, but not on account of public opprobrium. Rather than marking a recoil from animal experiments, Victoria's vivisection regulations of 1881 foreshadowed a largely unvoiced acquiescence to this new mode of epistemological sovereignty. Henceforth, professionalisation and sequestration would typify the local generation and global circulation of medical knowledge about snakes – and especially their venoms.

Notes

1 See for instance, Stefan Petrow, 'Civilizing mission: animal protection in Hobart 1878–1914', *Britain and the World*, 5:1 (2012), pp. 69–95; Jennifer MacCulloch, 'Creatures of culture: the animal protection and preservation movements in Sydney, 1880–1930' (PhD thesis, University of Sydney, 1993), pp. 18–91; R.B. Walker, 'Fauna and flora protection in New South Wales, 1866–1948', *Journal of Australian Studies*, 28 (1991), pp. 17–28.
2 Siobhan O'Sullivan, *Animals, Equality and Democracy* (Basingstoke: Palgrave Macmillan, 2012), p. 4.
3 See Arthur MacGregor, *Animal Encounters: Human and Animal Interaction in Britain from the Norman Conquest to World War One* (London: Reaktion Books, 2012), pp. 144–9, 215–22.
4 Harriet Ritvo, *The Platypus and the Mermaid and Other Figments of the Classifying Imagination* (Cambridge, Mass.: Harvard University Press, 1998), pp. 39, 191–4.
5 King James version.
6 Thomas R. Dunlap, *Nature and the English Diaspora: Environment and History in the United States, Canada, Australia, and New Zealand* (Cambridge: Cambridge University Press, 1999), pp. 80–1.
7 See Adrian Franklin, *Animal Nation: The True Story of Animals and Australia* (Sydney: University of New South Wales Press, 2006), pp. 107–15.
8 C.F.H. Jenkins, *The Noah's Ark Syndrome: One Hundred Years of Acclimatisation and Zoo Development in Australia* (Perth: Zoological Gardens Board of Western Australia, 1977), pp. 24, 94.
9 Kevin Markwell and Nancy Cushing, 'The "killer of the cane fields": the social

construction of the Australian coastal taipan', *Journal of Australian Studies*, 40:1 (2016), pp. 77, 89–90.

10 For example, Alexandra Minna Stern, 'Yellow fever crusade: US colonialism, tropical medicine, and the international politics of mosquito control, 1900–1920', in Alison Bashford (ed.), *Medicine at the Border: Disease, Globalization and Security, 1850 to the Present* (Houndmills: Palgrave Macmillan, 2006), pp. 41–59; Heather Schell, 'Tiger tales', in Deborah Denenholz Morse and Martin A. Danahay (eds), *Victorian Animal Dreams: Representations of Animals in Victorian Literature and Culture* (Aldershot: Ashgate, 2007), pp. 230–48.

11 Ada Cambridge, '(Arriving in Melbourne)', in Elizabeth Webby (ed.), *Colonial Voices: Letters, Diaries, Journalism and Other Accounts of Nineteenth-Century Australia* (St Lucia: University of Queensland Press, 1989), p. 47.

12 Kathleen Fitzpatrick, *Sir John Franklin in Tasmania 1837–1843* (Melbourne: Melbourne University Press, 1949), pp. 41–2. For records of the bounty scheme, see State Library of New South Wales, Sydney (hereafter SLNSW), A593, James Erskine Calder, 'Papers relating to snakes in Tasmania'.

13 Joyce Westrip and Peggy Holroyde, *Colonial Cousins: A Surprising History of Connections between India and Australia* (Kent Town: Wakefield Press, 2010), pp. 306–12; Michael James Slouber, 'Gāruda medicine: a history of snakebite and religious healing in South Asia' (PhD thesis, University of California, 2012), pp. 107–9.

14 For instance, see Barbara Pertzel, *For All Creatures: A History of RSPCA Victoria* (Burwood East: RSPCA Victoria, 2006), pp. 10, 27; Wallace B. Budd, *Hear the Other Side: The R.S.P.C.A. in South Australia, 1875–1988* (Hawthorndene: Investigator Press, 1988), pp. 30–1, 167; Stefan Petrow, '"Developing the highest moral instincts": protecting animals in Launceston 1879–1906', *History Australia*, 15:3 (2015), pp. 160–82.

15 Daniel Gilfoyle, 'Veterinary research and the African rinderpest epizootic: the Cape Colony, 1896–1898', *Journal of Southern African Studies*, 29:1 (2003), pp. 133–54.

16 Karen Brown, *Mad Dogs and Meerkats: A History of Resurgent Rabies in Southern Africa* (Cape Town: University of Cape Town Press, 2011), pp. 46–50.

17 Victorian Society for the Protection of Animals, *A Few Words to Young Australians* (Melbourne: Victorian Society for the Protection of Animals, 1883), p. 3.

18 Richard D. French, *Antivivisection and Medical Science in Victorian Society* (Princeton: Princeton University Press, 1975), pp. 232–3.

19 James Turner, *Reckoning with the Beast: Animals, Pain and Humanity in the Victorian Mind* (Baltimore: Johns Hopkins University Press, 1980), pp. 45, 115–17.

20 Anita Guerrini, *Experimenting with Humans and Animals: From Galen to Animal Rights* (Baltimore: Johns Hopkins University Press, 2003), p. 89.

21 Victoria, *An Act for the Protection of Animals*, 45 Vict. 712 (24 December 1881), pp. 1, 3. Punctuation as per the original.

22 *Ibid.*, p. 3.

23 Craig Buettinger, 'Women and antivivisection in late nineteenth-century America', *Journal of Social History*, 30:4 (1997), pp. 858, 866–7; Patricia Peck Gossel, 'William Henry Welch and the antivivisection legislation in the District of Columbia, 1896–1900', *Journal of the History of Medicine and Allied Sciences*, 40:4 (1985), pp. 405–17; Karen D. Ross, 'Recruiting "friends of medical progress": evolving tactics in the defense of animal experimentation, 1910s and 1920s', *Journal of the History of Medicine and Allied Sciences*, 70:3 (2015), pp. 367–70.

24 French, *Antivivisection and Medical Science in Victorian Society*, p. 41.

25 Diana Manuel, 'Marshall Hall (1790–1857): vivisection and the development of experimental physiology', in Nicolaas Rupke (ed.) *Vivisection in Historical Perspective* (London: Croom Helm, 1987), pp. 85–7.

26 Stewart Richards, 'Vicarious suffering, necessary pain: physiological method in late nineteenth-century Britain', in Nicolaas Rupke (ed.) *Vivisection in Historical Perspective* (London: Croom Helm, 1987), pp. 134–9.

27 United Kingdom, *An Act to Amend the Law Relating to Cruelty to Animals*, 39 & 40 Vict. c. 77 (15 August 1876), sections 5, 10.

28 Paul S. White, 'The experimental animal in Victorian Britain', in Lorraine Daston and Gregg Mitman (eds), *Thinking with Animals: New Perspectives on Anthropomorphism* (New York: Columbia University Press, 2005), p. 62.

29 See Michael A. Finn, and James F. Stark, 'Medical science and the Cruelty to Animals Act 1876: a re-examination of anti-vivisectionism in provincial Britain', *Studies in History and Philosophy of Science Part C: Studies in History and Philosophy of Biological and Biomedical Sciences*, 49 (2015), pp. 12–23.

30 Nicolaas Rupke, 'Introduction', in Nicolaas Rupke (ed.), *Vivisection in Historical Perspective* (London: Croom Helm, 1987), pp. 7–8.

31 See E.M. Tansey, 'The Wellcome Physiological Research Laboratories 1894–1904: the Home Office, pharmaceutical firms, and animal experiments', *Medical History*, 33:1 (1989), pp. 5–11, 19–41.

32 Victorian Society for the Prevention of Cruelty to Animals, *Man's Duty To the Lower Animals: Especially Addressed to Victorians* (Melbourne: Mason, Firth & McCutcheon, 1880), p. 3. Italics in original.

33 *Victoria. Parliamentary Debates. Session 1881. Legislative Council and Legislative Assembly* (Melbourne: John Ferres, 1882), p. 245.

34 *Ibid.*, p. 344. Melbourne University's Professor of Natural History, Frederick McCoy, appears never to have conducted experiments upon live animals – not even snakes.

35 *Ibid.*, p. 897.

36 Philip Jamieson, 'Duty and the beast: the movement in reform of animal welfare law', *University of Queensland Law Journal*, 16:2 (1991), p. 243. See also United Kingdom, *An Act to Amend the Law Relating to Cruelty to Animals*, 1876, section 3 and 'Administration of Law', section 3.

37 Public Records Office of Victoria, Melbourne (hereafter PROV), VPRS 1676 Unit 3, Chief Secretary's Office: Record of Licences and Warrants Issued – Record Book No. 23, 1882–91.

38 Helen MacDonald, *Possessing the Dead: The Artful Science of Anatomy* (Melbourne: Melbourne University Press, 2010), p. 170.

39 United Kingdom, *An Act to Amend the Law Relating to Cruelty to Animals*, 1876, section 6.

40 Benjamin Bryan (ed.), *The Vivisectors' Directory: Being a List of the Licensed Vivisectors in the United Kingdom, Together with the Leading Physiologists in Foreign Laboratories* (London: Victoria Street Society for the Protection of Animals from Vivisection, United with the International Association for the Total Suppression of Vivisection, 1884), *passim*.

41 French, *Antivivisection and Medical Science in Victorian Society*, p. 334.

42 PROV 1676 Unit 3, pp. 30, 39; James Barrett, *Eighty Eventful Years* (Melbourne: J.C. Stephens, 1945), pp. 28–9.

43 D. McAlpine, 'Observations on the movements of the heart of the copper-head snake (*Hoplocephalus superbus*, Günth.) in and out of the body', *Proceedings of the Royal Society of Victoria*, 3 (1891), pp. 28–31, 34.

44 PROV VPRS 1187 Unit 64 (K), Chief Secretary's Office: Outward Letter Book – 29 May 1883 to 3 October 1883, TR Wilson to GB Halford, 27 September 1883, pp. 1–2.

45 PROV VPRS 1187 Unit 70 (R), Chief Secretary's Office: Outward Letter Book – 30 April 1885 to 15 September 1885, Under Secretary to The Inspector, Society for Protection of Animals, 25 August 1885.

46 University of Melbourne Archives, Melbourne, 1981.0062, Halford, George Britton, 'Letters responding to appeal for snakes heads – Aug–Sept 1894', John Madden to George Halford, 15 October 1894, p. 2.

47 For instance, Victorian Society for the Protection of Animals, *Twelfth Annual Report* (Melbourne: Victorian Society for the Protection of Animals, 1883); Archives Office of Tasmania, Hobart, NS647/1/1, Minutes, annual reports and press reports of the Southern Branch of the RSPCA, 'Minutes of meetings of the

Committee of the Society', 1889–1914; State Library of Victoria, Melbourne, Australian Association against Painful Experiments on Animals, 'Press cuttings and other items', 1874–1976.

48 These Acts were not revised until 1977–85: Jamieson, 'Duty and the beast', p. 249.

49 A. Mueller, 'On the action of snake-poison and the use of strychnine as an antidote', *Australian Medical Journal*, 10 (1888), p. 200.

50 A. Mueller, 'A contribution to the history of medicine in Australia', *Australasian Medical Gazette*, 9 (1890), p. 153.

51 'The hypodermic injection of strychnia in snakebite', *Australasian Medical Gazette*, 10 (1890), p. 91. See also SLNSW, A 694, John Mildred Creed – papers 1882–1911, Augustus Mueller to John Mildred Creed, 14 September 1888 and 4 May 1890.

52 François Magendie, *Formulary for the Preparation and Employment of Several New Remedies*, 6th edn, trans. Joseph Houlton (London: T. and G. Underwood, 1829), p. 19.

53 David Arnold, 'The politics of poison: healing, empowerment and subversion in nineteenth-century India', in David Hardiman and Projit Bihari Mukharji (eds), *Medical Marginality in South Asia: Situating Subaltern Therapeutics* (Abingdon: Routledge, 2012), p. 171.

54 See John Buckingham, *Bitter Nemesis: The Intimate History of Strychnine* (Boca Raton: CRC Press, 2008), pp. 154–7, 202–5; Raymond Evans, '"Plenty shoot 'em": the destruction of Aboriginal societies along the Queensland frontier', in A. Dirk Moses (ed.), *Genocide and Settler Society: Frontier Violence and Stolen Indigenous Children in Australian History* (New York: Berghahn Books, 2004), p. 158.

55 See John Pearn, '"Where there is no doctor": self-help and pre-hospital care in colonial Australia', *Health and History*, 14:2 (2012), pp. 162–80.

56 'The medicines most used. An analysis of seven thousand prescriptions', *Chemist and Druggist of Australasia*, 16:2 (1901), p. 67.

57 'Intercolonial Medical Congress of Australasia. Second session', *Chemist and Druggist of Australasia*, 4:2 (1889), pp. 54–9. See also SLNSW A 694, Augustus Mueller to John Mildred Creed, 18 March 1892, pp. 1–2.

58 Mueller, 'A contribution to the history of medicine in Australia', p. 153.

59 Roy MacLeod, 'Organizing science under the Southern Cross', in Roy MacLeod (ed.), *The Commonwealth of Science: ANZAAS and the Scientific Enterprise in Australasia, 1888–1988* (Melbourne: Oxford University Press, 1988), pp. 24–35; Colin Finney, *Paradise Revealed: Natural History in Nineteenth-Century Australia* (Melbourne: Museum of Victoria, 1993), pp. 136–41.

60 Augustus Mueller, 'On the pathology and cure of snake-bite. II', *Australasian Medical Gazette*, 8 (1888), p. 68.

61 Augustus Mueller, 'On the pathology and cure of snake-bite. IV', *Australasian Medical Gazette*, 8 (1889), p. 181.

62 A. Mueller, 'Snake-poison; its physical and chemical qualities and physiological action', in L. Ralston Huxtable (ed.), *Intercolonial Medical Congress of Australasia. Transactions of the Third Session, Held in Sydney, New South Wales, September, 1892* (Sydney: Charles Potter, 1893), p. 161.

63 Mueller, 'On the action of snake-poison and the use of strychnine as an antidote', p. 204.

64 A. Mueller, 'Dr. A. Feoktistow's experimental researches on snake poison', *Australasian Medical Gazette*, 8 (1889), pp. 283–4.

65 Sharon Louise Wallace, 'Treatment of snakebite from Halford to Sutherland' (BMedSci thesis, University of Melbourne, 1983), p. 59.

66 John V. Pickstone, 'Museological science? The place of the analytical/comparative in nineteenth-century science, technology and medicine', *History of Science*, 32:2 (1994), pp. 117–18, 130–3.

67 Ohad Parnes, 'From agents to cells: Theodor Schwann's research notes of the years

1835–1838', in Frederic L. Holmes, Jürgen Renn, and Hans-Jörg Rheinberger (eds), *Reworking the Bench: Research Notebooks in the History of Science* (Dordrecht: Kluwer Academic, 2003), p. 125.

68 G. Hogarth Pringle, 'The blood in snake-poisoning', *Australian Medical Journal*, 13 (1868), p. 286; V. Richards, 'Experiments with strychnine as an antidote to snake-poison', *Medical Times and Gazette*, 1 (1874), p. 595.

69 Augustus Mueller, 'On the pathology and cure of snakebite. V', *Australasian Medical Gazette*, 8 (1889), p. 209.

70 Ana Carolina Vimieiro Gomes, '"Too good to be true": the controversy over the use of permanganate of potash as an antidote to snake poison and the circulation of Brazilian physiology in the nineteenth century', *Bulletin of the History of Medicine*, 86:2 (2012), pp. 164, 176.

71 John Bennett, 'Strychnine in snakebite', *Australasian Medical Gazette*, 13 (1894), p. 359.

72 'Strychnine in snake-bite', *Australasian Medical Gazette*, 10 (1891), p. 243.

73 C.H. Campbell, 'Dr. Mueller's strychnine cure of snake-bite', *Medical Journal of Australia*, 2 (1968), pp. 4–5.

74 A. Mueller, 'On haematuria in snakebite poisoning', *Australasian Medical Gazette*, 12 (1893), p. 249.

75 Augustus Mueller, 'Special communication', *Journal of the Transactions of the Victoria Institute, or Philosophical Society of Great Britain*, 26 (1893), p. 120.

76 Iwan Rhys Morus, 'Worlds of wonder: sensation and the Victorian scientific performance', *Isis*, 101:4 (2010), p. 816.

77 Richard Rendle, *Notes on Snake Bite. Full Directions, What to Do, What to Avoid, and How to Use the Strychnia Antidote, Together With a Description of Queensland Venomous Snakes and How to Distinguish the Venomous from the Harmless*, 2nd edn (Brisbane: Pole, Outridge and Co., 1892), p. 18.

78 'Strychnine in snake-bite', *Chemist and Druggist of Australasia*, 7:1 (1892), p. 4.

79 'Applications for patents', *Victoria Government Gazette*, 63 (12 May 1891), p. 1981.

80 A. Mueller, *On Snake-Poison. Its Action and Its Antidote* (Sydney: L. Bruck, 1893), p. 62.

81 Stanley Joel Reiser, *Medicine and the Reign of Technology* (Cambridge: Cambridge University Press, 1978), p. 90.

82 Robert G. Frank, 'The telltale heart: physiological instruments, graphic methods, and clinical hopes 1854–1914', in William Coleman and Frederic L. Holmes (eds), *The Investigative Enterprise: Experimental Physiology in Nineteenth-Century Medicine* (Berkeley: University of California Press, 1988), pp. 211–90.

83 'Snake poison and its antidote', *Chemist and Druggist of Australasia*, 8:7 (1893), p. 147.

84 J.M. Creed, 'New South Wales Branch of the British Medical Association. Presidential address', *Australasian Medical Gazette*, 12 (1893), p. 151.

85 State Records Office of Western Australia, Perth, 1892/078 Consignment 1218, Deaths from snake or insect bite – return 1881 to 1891 – asks for, L Ralston Huxtable to the Government Statistician, 12 May 1892.

86 See also 'Snake-bite in Australia – recent statistics, and a review of recent observations', *Chemist and Druggist of Australasia*, 8:5 (1893), p. 103.

87 L. Ralston Huxtable, 'Snake-bite in Australia – recent statistics and a review of recent observations', in L. Ralston Huxtable (ed.), *Intercolonial Medical Congress of Australasia. Transactions of the Third Session, Held in Sydney, New South Wales, September, 1892* (Sydney: Charles Potter, 1893), pp. 142–4.

88 James W. Barrett, 'The present position of the snake-bite controversy', *Proceedings of the Royal Society of Victoria*, 5 (1893), pp. 185–6.

89 Mueller, *On Snake-Poison*, pp. 10–12. See Gael Phillips, 'Snakebite remedies: an historical review of snake bite management in the Australian outback', in John Pearn (ed.), *Outback Medicine: Some Vignettes of Pioneering Medicine* (Brisbane: Amphion Press, 1994), pp. 76–80.

90 A. Müller, 'Ueber die behandlung des schlangenbisses durch strychnin', *Virchows Archiv für Pathologische Anatomie und Physiologie und für Klinische Medizin*, 113:2 (1888), p. 393.

91 Dr Macher, 'The use of strychnine in snake-bite', trans. H.H. Behr, *Therapeutic Gazette*, 18:8 (1894), p. 519.

92 Leonhard Stejneger, *The Poisonous Snakes of North America* (Washington: Government Printing Office, 1895), p. 469. Italics in original.

93 SLNSW A 694, Victor Child-Villiers to John Mildred Creed, 5 March 1892.

94 'Strychnine in snakebite', *Australasian Medical Gazette*, 12 (1893), p. 27.

95 Joshua Duke, 'The symptoms and treatment of snake-bite in India, with special mention of Dr. A. Mueller's subcutaneous injection of strychnine, based on the consideration of 37 cases', *Indian Medical Gazette*, 30:6 (1895), p. 209.

96 R.P. Banerjee, 'The hypodermic use of strychnine in cases of Indian snakebite', *Australasian Medical Gazette*, 11 (1892), p. 293; Thos. L. Bancroft, 'Strychnine in snakebite', *Australasian Medical Gazette*, 12 (1893), p. 384.

97 R.P. Banerjee, 'A reply from India to the opponents of strychnine treatment in snakebite', *Australasian Medical Gazette*, 11 (1892), p. 388.

98 J.H. Tull Walsh, '"On Snake-Poison: Its Action and Its Antidote" by A.M. Mueller, M.D., L. Bruck, Sydney', *Indian Medical Gazette*, 28:9 (1893), p. 324.

99 J. Duke, 'The symptoms and treatment of snake bite in India with special mention of Dr. A. Mueller's subcutaneous injection of strychnine, based on the consideration of 37 cases', in Robert Bird (ed.), *Transactions of the First Indian Medical Congress Held at St. Xavier's College, Calcutta, 24th to 29th December, 1894* (Calcutta: Caledonian Steam Printing Works, 1895), p. 495.

100 I have been unable to obtain the original article, viz. R.H. Elliot, 'Is strychnine an antidote to cobra poison?' *Transactions of the South Indian Branch of the British Medical Association* 2 (1894), n.p.

101 'Strychnine as an antidote to cobra poison', *British Medical Journal*, 1:1790 (1895), p. 884.

102 D.D. Cunningham, 'Salts of strychnia as remedies for snake-bite', in Robert Bird (ed.), *Transactions of the First Indian Medical Congress held at St. Xavier's College, Calcutta, 24*th *to 29*th *December, 1894* (Calcutta: Caledonian Steam Printing Works, 1895), p. 489.

103 A. Mueller, 'Discoursive notes on snake poison and the strychnine treatment', *Indian Medical Record*, 8 (1895), pp. 54–5.

104 John William Springthorpe, *Therapeutics, Dietetics and Hygiene: An Australian Text-book* (Melbourne: James Little, 1914), p. 872. Italics in original.

105 Frank Tidswell, *Researches on Australian Venoms. Snake-Bite, Snake-Venom and Antivenine. The Poison of the Platypus. The Poison of the Red-Spotted Spider* (Sydney: William Applegate Gullick, 1906), pp. 21, 39, 41. Calculations corrected from data in the text.

106 William Murrell, *What to Do in Cases of Poisoning* (London: HK Lewis & Co, 1921), p. 201; *Pharmacopœia and Reference Handbook of the Royal Alexandria Hospital for Children, Sydney*, 8th edn (Sydney: Australasian Medical Publishing Company, 1951), pp. 88–9.

107 For instance, Campbell, 'Dr. Mueller's strychnine cure of snake-bite', p. 6; Wallace, 'Treatment of snakebite from Halford to Sutherland', p. 56.

108 See Christoph Gradmann, 'Locating therapeutic vaccines in nineteenth-century history', *Science in Context*, 21:2 (2008), pp. 145–60.

CHAPTER SIX

Immunology and indigeneity: species, serums and localisms, 1890–1914

The quantitative turn in pathology, bacteriology and physiology after 1880 has generated a robust historiography. At its crux lie conjoint questions of scientific authority and professional testimony, centred upon novel technologies which established ontological agents as prima facie causes of disease.[1] Yet these clinical innovations – including Listerian antisepsis, Kochian bacteriology, vaccines and serum therapy – entailed a substantial but frequently submerged animal sacrifice.

Horses in particular, note Axel Hüntelmann and Jonathan Simon, became favoured 'units of serum production', monitored not for their welfare but to maximise exploitation of their standardised immunological labour.[2] Yet as Michael Lynch and Ilana Löwy have shown, the idiosyncrasies of individual animals insistently shaped the praxis, potency and knowledge claims of early biomedicine.[3] Universalism was likewise challenged by the particularities of place, insists Pratik Chakrabarti. With antivivisection campaigns constraining serum harvesting and testing in Britain, it was precisely by arrogating to themselves a moral ascendancy that Raj doctors and administrators 'consistently projected Indian social practices as the main sites of cruelty rather than the laboratories'.[4]

Snakes also proved central to this *fin de siècle* iteration of 'scientific medicine', in turn comprising exemplars and victims of its ontological transformations. In the Australian colonies, which federated in 1901, venoms complemented bacterial pathogens as models for the emerging field of immunology. Yet like the serum drained from experimental guinea pigs or 'industrialised' horses – or indeed the advent of pooled and pasteurised cows' milk – serology largely parsed venom from its animal origins.[5]

Bringing animals into newly instrumented laboratories flattened their moral status and denied their autonomy. If in 1894 Sydney

University's Dean of Medicine, Thomas Anderson Stuart, outlined this emerging epistemology by asserting that it was 'not enough to cause a snake to bite an animal, and merely stand by and observe what happens', George Halford encapsulated its new mode.[6] He requested that Australians fuel research not by supplying snakes, but merely their decapitated heads.[7]

Through the 1890s, vivisection proved pivotal to successive variants of 'scientific medicine' targeting snakebite, yet only one changed quotidian medical practice. John Pickstone and Michael Worboys urge stepping back from scientific novelties to 'give a better sense of the synchronic assemblages of practices and hybrid knowledges ... [that] help indicate how mundane activities change'.[8] One such mundanity remained animal experimentation, which severed not only direct contact between snake and victim, but between snakes and their own venoms (Figure 25). This particularisation ultimately proved self-defeating. By elaborating the complexity of venoms, immunology and physiological chemistry dismissed the possibility of a universal antidote for snakebite. Indeed, advancing highly specific antivenenes proved a clinical dead end, defeated by the variable character of the snakes themselves.

Dogs, ticks and guinea pigs

In the *British Medical Journal*'s first article for 1891, Thomas Lauder Brunton – the Empire's pre-eminent pharmacologist – ventured a new mode of therapy. After reading snakebite reports in the Indian medical press, he invoked American physiologist Henry Sewall, who in 1887 claimed to have rendered pigeons 'immune' to rattlesnake venom by inoculating them with small but increasing doses.[9] Perhaps, proposed Brunton, 'the system may gradually become resistant to the action of snake venom, just as it may to that of infective diseases such as anthrax ... the analogies between it and the products of disease germs are becoming every day more apparent'.[10]

Venoms were foundational to the novel field of immunology, yet their role is frequently sidelined. If not quite accurate in asserting that 'snake venom research was indistinguishable from late nineteenth- and early twentieth-century bacteriology', Chakrabarti is correct in proposing that these endeavours were united by dreams of creating 'a universal panacea against a local scourge'.[11] The concept of developing constitutional hardiness via exposure to small quantities of poison dated to antiquity, being regularly invoked to explain why snake charmers apparently resisted envenomation (see Chapter 2). Throughout the nineteenth century, variolation and vaccination

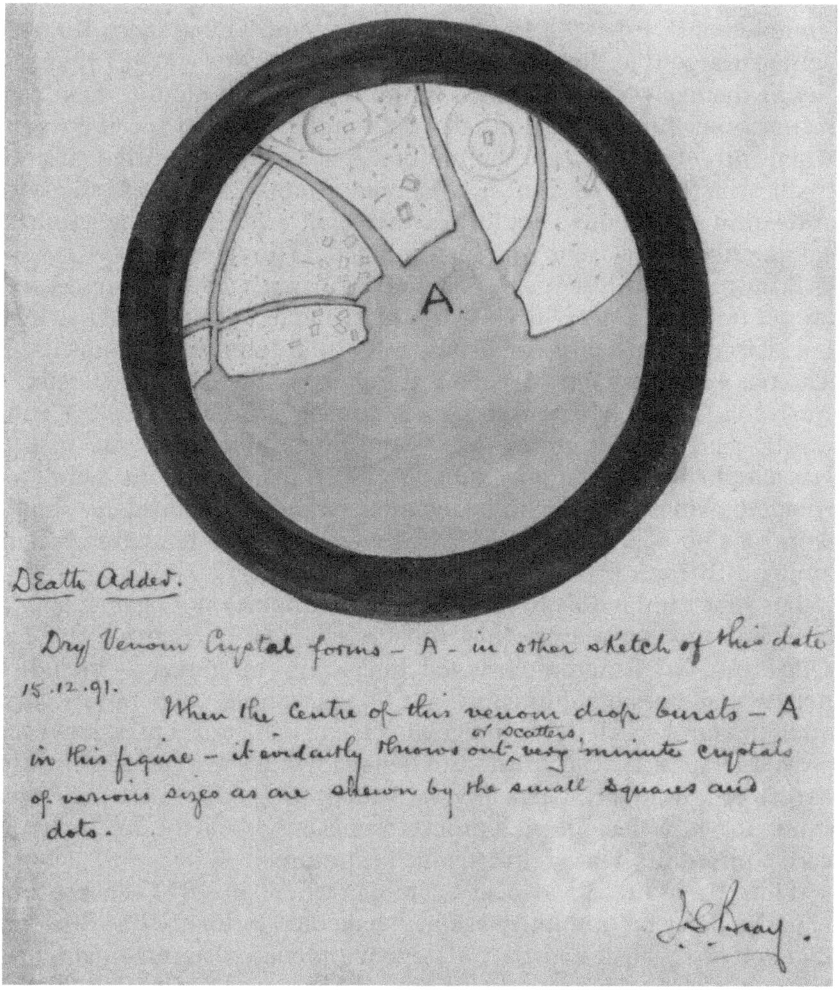

25 James S. Bray, 'Death adder', 15 December 1891.

institutionalised a belief that prophylactic exposure to contagious matter *might* prevent more severe manifestations. Smallpox, however, remained a prominent outlier until the early 1880s, when Louis Pasteur trumpeted vaccines against fowl cholera, anthrax and rabies.

United by ontological conceptions of disease aetiology, from 1888 immunological investigators were divided by mechanism. Pasteur Institute worker Élie Metchnikoff propounded a cellular theory: circulating phagocytes assailed foreign substances. Humoralists argued that blood serum itself contained an active antitoxic principle, later termed 'complement'. By 1890, Emil von Behring and Shibasaburo Kitasato demonstrated that diphtheria and tetanus exotoxins – rather than the bacilli themselves – stimulated immunity. Their announcement that serum from immunised animals could protect against specific toxins when introduced into another animal – or human – spurred an anti-toxin arms race.[12] As Pauline Mazumdar remarks, the specificity of antiserum soon defined not just its therapeutic value, but the ontological identity of the agent which stimulated its production.[13]

Brunton's 1891 leader also coincided with early antipodean research on neutralising animal toxins. In Queensland, ophthalmologist John Lockhart Gibson discussed inducing immunity to venoms with Thomas Lane Bancroft. Arguably the most skilled pharmacologist in Australia, Bancroft never treated a human snakebite case.[14] Citing results generated in guinea pigs – the first time this exotic species was employed for venom studies in Australia – Bancroft dismissed Augustus Mueller's strychnine injection, arguing that antidotes should work not by opposing physiological effects, but by rendering venom biologically inert.[15]

His first gambit was to induce active immunity not against snake-bite, but tick poisoning. In a long-overlooked 1891 article in *The Queenslander*, Bancroft observed that many mammals – including horses and possibly humans – were susceptible to paralysis after attachment of scrub ticks. Indigenous fauna and guinea pigs, however, proved inherently resistant to tick poison, which was 'probably of the nature of a ferment'. Critically, he stated, 'Dogs that have recovered from tick bite become tick-proof', proposing a scheme for inducing active immunity via carefully graded exposure.[16]

Thus Bancroft had a local exemplar when, in 1892, he contemplated generating immunity against snakebite. Influenced by Brunton, Bancroft first suggested that a serpent's blood or serum might neutralise its venom. He found that black snakes possessed a remarkable immunity to their own venom, suggesting an antidotal substance within their tissues. Further experiments saw him abandon this theory, arguing instead that low blood temperature allowed serpents to resist envenomation.[17] Concurrently, Bancroft injected escalating doses of venom into guinea pigs. 'Judging from the success obtained by the use of the serum of animals immune to tetanus', he insisted, citing Gibson's bacteriological research, 'it is reasonable to hope that the serum of animals immune to snake venom might prove useful as a remedy in snake-bite'.[18]

Rarely lauded for his tenacity, by 1894 Bancroft had passed the baton to another expert who likened snake venom to bacterial toxins. Thomas Fraser, Dean of the University of Edinburgh's Medical Faculty, rivalled Brunton as a doyen of experimental pharmacology and toxicology. At first dismissing acquired resistance to snakebite as mere tribal superstition, Fraser was apparently convinced by Bancroft's suggestion that poisonous snakes were immune to their own venom. 'The relationship of such observations to the recent discoveries in connection with the toxines of Tetanus, Diphtheria and other diseases', he professed, 'could not long remain unrecognised.'[19]

By 1895 Fraser had generated active immunity against snake venoms. His global network supplied samples from Indian cobras, American rattlesnakes, African rinkhals (spitting cobras) and 'a large unidentified snake of the Diamantina district of South Australia'.[20] Reviewing his vast experience with poisons, Fraser asserted that cobra venom 'takes a position among the most active of known substances' – although the Australian venom quietly occupied second place. Slowly escalating successive inoculations, he claimed to protect rabbits against 50 lethal doses of Indian cobra venom. 'There are few facts in the whole range of biology', he exclaimed, 'more calculated to arrest the attention or produce astonishment in the mind of the observer!'[21]

Fraser's experiments furthermore suggested that animals immunised against one serpent's venom became less susceptible to others. His Scottish rabbits thus became the first individuals in history poisoned in succession by American, Australian and Indian snakes. Questioning whether the blood of animals immunised against venom might rescue envenomed humans, Fraser quoted Bancroft's similar hypothesis.[22] He used samples supplied by Bancroft to demonstrate in rabbits that Australian black snake venom could be neutralised by first admixing it with serum from the same serpent. This protection, however, was not of the order obtained by immunising rabbits with Indian cobra venom.

Indeed, Fraser's novel therapeutic proved as astonishingly potent as the poison. It could prevent death when administered up to 30 minutes after envenomation – even with different venoms. Because it acted not as a physiological antagonist like strychnine, but directly neutralised venom in an apparently stoichiometric chemical relationship, Fraser neologised. 'To this serum, whether in the dry form or in solution, it would be convenient to apply the name "*antivenene*".'[23] In mid-1895, samples generated in a horse at Edinburgh's New Veterinary College were despatched to treat snakebites in India and Africa. 'Against this ever-present and formidable enemy', he deigned, 'the inhabitants of these countries have awaited for centuries a remedy whose antidotal value and limits of curative power have been established by experimental demonstration'.[24] Beleaguered Australians, apparently, were left unprotected.

It would be erroneous to assert that Fraser and Bancroft generated a new therapeutic paradigm. Nevertheless, two important developments emerged through this neglected Queensland–Scotland collaboration. First, Bancroft's method exemplified a new mode of colonial experimental medicine: remoteness from clinical practice and reliance on theorisation and vivisection. Second, Fraser's term 'antivenene' proved telling. No longer were snakes, or even snakebite, targets for therapeutic intervention. Exemplified by Fraser's dried samples circuiting the globe, venoms themselves were now fully autonomous actants.

Asian antivenin: the Pasteur product, 1895–1900

As Fraser himself acknowledged, his antivenene was preceded by a French *antivenin*. In 1891, the Pasteur Institute of Cochin-China was established in Saigon, primarily as a commercial venture to investigate tropical diseases and produce vaccines against endemic smallpox and rabies.[25] The arrival of a barrelful of live cobras, however, coincided with an Indian Government reward for devising a novel snakebite remedy. The new director of l'Institut en petit – Albert Calmette – began to explore neutralising cobra venom. As a serpent dreaded across Asia, mastering cobra bites would represent a civilising achievement for *médecin colonial* almost as worthy as conquering tropical fevers (Figure 26).

After investigating chemical approaches, early in 1894 Calmette attempted immunisation. Inducing immunity to lethal doses in guinea pigs and rabbits, inoculation with cobra venom subsequently seemed

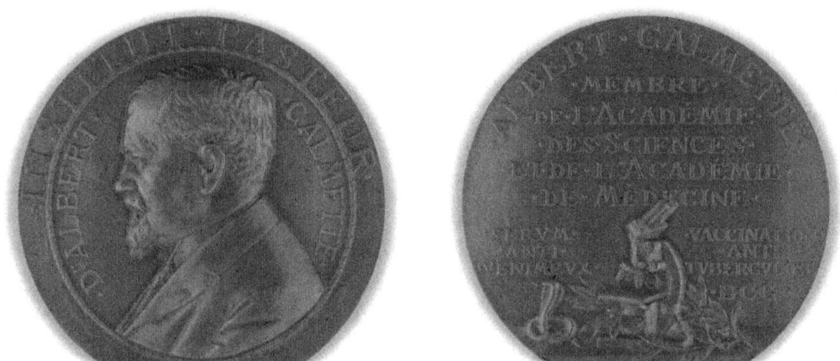

26 Pasteur Institute medal commemorating the contributions of Albert Calmette to tropical medicine and immunology.

to confer resistance against the venoms of *all* snakes. The mechanism, he explained, was identical to that which rendered animals impervious to tetanus and diphtheria toxins. Unlike Fraser, Calmette did not suggest that *antivenin* directly inactivated venom; rather, he followed his Pasteur Institute colleague Metchnikoff in believing that the antitoxin rendered the victim's cells less susceptible to poison. From the outset he foresaw the commercial potential of saving human and animal lives wherever venomous serpents abounded – including India and Australia.[26]

Following the serum standardisation methods of Behring, (Pierre) Émile Roux and Louis Vaillard, Calmette was obliged to establish minimum lethal doses of venoms in rabbits. Just as Fraser had found, Australian serpents suddenly ascended to an unimagined potency, second only to the cobra. Among his samples were Australian tiger snake venom, which arrived via Albert Dastre, professor of physiology at the Sorbonne, while Émile Roux at the Pasteur Institute forwarded black snake samples that had, in turn, reached France courtesy of Sydneysider John McGarvie Smith.[27] In Melbourne, the ageing Halford now appealed for decapitated serpent heads, intending to forward them to Calmette in the ironic hope that 'a great reciprocal work will be commenced between India [*sic*] and Australia'.[28]

Trading on the Pasteurian model of applied investigation and aggressively commercialised therapeutics, Calmette's curative serum constituted the last word in medical modernity. Early in 1895 he supervised production of *Serum Antivenimeux anglicé Antivenine* by mixing cobra and viper venoms in an 80:20 ratio, heating and filtering the hybrid, then inoculating it into monkeys, donkeys and 'cobra horses'.[29] Seeking to prove its universal efficacy, his venom range now included samples from the Australian death adder and broad-headed snake – again provided by Smith via Roux – further elevating antipodean venoms in global toxicity rankings.

This diversity of samples did not lessen Calmette's ambitions. In August 1896 he was invited to London to demonstrate *Serum Antivenimeux* before a Conjoint Board of the Royal Colleges of Physicians and Surgeons. Convincingly rescuing European rabbits from Indian cobra venom, he boasted that 'after many experiments I succeeded some time ago in placing in the hands of doctors in India and Australia a serum, the value of which has now been proved in a small number of cases' – although none hailed from Australia. Ever-prepared, he proposed that 'stations provided with serum and all the necessary apparatus for its application be established in … the Colonies infested with venomous snakes, such as Australia, Burmah, and India, so that every person bitten may be able to come at once and receive treatment'.[30]

The Imperial hubris was patent. Rather than colonists equipping themselves with pocket-cases, snakebite therapy would be medicalised, centralised, standardised, supervised and – presumably – subsidised by the state. It was not to be. If Pasteur himself had in 1888 imagined 'a single factory' in Sydney which would supply vaccines for the entire continent, by 1896 the Pasteur Institute's gambit was dashed against the biological complexity of Australian snake venoms.[31]

Bovines and bacilli: Australian embrace of vaccines and serums

By the mid-1890s, Australians were surprisingly receptive to immunological innovation, especially in the democratic arena of commercial sales. Biological agents were not new to the colonies: in 1853 Victoria and South Australia joined the UK in passing Compulsory Vaccination Acts, followed by Van Diemen's Land in 1854, Western Australia in 1860 and New Zealand in 1863. As contentious in the antipodes as in Britain, these laws were enforced with waning degrees of conviction; neither New South Wales nor Queensland ever enacted equivalent legislation.[32]

This is not to suggest that smallpox vaccination 'failed' in the antipodes. First imported into New South Wales in 1804 and Van Diemen's Land the following year, British vaccine lymph was supplemented by cowpox introduced into Hobart in 1841 and, from 1847, Sydney's Vaccine Institute. Transitioning to calf lymph in 1882 – using material from government sources in Australia, New Zealand and occasionally India – interspecies tensions underlying bovinised vaccines persisted, as Alison Bashford demonstrates.[33] Yet even as local antivaccinationist agitation grew from 1880, clinicians embraced the practice as emblematic of medical orthodoxy.

Animals, nevertheless, proved the vanguard for Australian adoption of immunology. Rabbits were doubtless the most prominent animal question plaguing late Victorian Australia. Commencing in 1888, an Intercolonial Royal Commission on Rabbit Destruction offered a munificent £25,000 prize, attracting numerous proposals from local and international venturers – including Pasteur. Indeed, his first facility beyond France was established at Rodd Island on Sydney Harbour in 1890.[34] The Pasteur Institute of Australia proposed passaged fowl cholera for rabbit destruction, although it was ultimately dismissed by the Commissioners. Its second product proved more profitable: veterinary vaccination against anthrax.[35] As Jan Todd details, despite Pasteur's infamous insistence on controlling production, a combination of parochialism, pragmatism and industrial espionage saw local anthrax vaccines out-compete the French product by 1894.[36]

Unlike its Saigon equivalent, the Pasteur Institute of Australia did not overtly investigate snake venoms. Its presence, however, stimulated local interest in both physiological chemistry (biochemistry) and serum therapy. Central to this exchange was John McGarvie Smith, a University of Sydney science graduate who by 1890 had established a private laboratory in inner Sydney. Unlike Britain – or ostensibly Victoria – in New South Wales investigators could vivisect with little legal constraint, notwithstanding the colony's *Animals Infectious Diseases Act* 1888, which prohibited unlicensed persons from inoculating 'any wild or domestic animal with any noxious and infectious microbes'.[37] Despite Board of Health alarm at the public health implications, Smith was licensed to infect rabbits with typhoid, tuberculosis and anthrax. By 1892, pastoralist John Gunn received a similar dispensation to introduce infectious diseases into rabbits. Developing an anthrax vaccine rivalling the Pasteur offering, his tests encompassed 200 lambs and then 12,100 sheep.[38]

Over 1891–92, Smith attempted to create the first serum against Australian snake venoms. He turned initially to Oscar Katz, a German microbiologist trained by Robert Koch but possessed of dubious skills. In 1888 Katz became the first investigator to publicly propose creating an Australian antivenene when, at the instigation of science patron William Macleay, he commenced desultory venom experiments. Probably having read Sewall's 1887 paper, key amongst Katz's questions was 'whether animals can be rendered immune from snakebite by previous inoculation with minute quantities of venom from the same or another species'.[39] Perhaps stimulated by Katz, Smith's immunisation of rabbits faltered, so he turned to Louis Momont, senior researcher and ultimately director on Rodd Island. The Frenchman avoided divulging Calmette's *antivenin* secrets, but offered Smith a position at the Institute; little wonder that he proved so eager to ship Australian venoms to Paris.

When Gunn and Smith subsequently partnered to develop a local anthrax vaccine, their immunological studies paralleled early European experiments with diphtheria antitoxin, which by 1900 symbolised the shining hope of serum therapy.[40] Although immunisation and antitoxins were united by the often distasteful notion of injecting animal products into human bodies, equally critical was the difference in observable outcomes.[41] While difficult to prove that vaccination prevented smallpox in individuals, the clinical results of injecting ailing patients with diphtheria antitoxin or *Serum Antivenimeux* were often immediate. Paul Weindling has elaborated how early European experience with diphtheria antitoxin revealed difficulties in standardising activity and appropriate dosing, stymying its clinical and public embrace.[42] In Australia, spectacular recoveries had already proved critical to the widespread adoption of both intravenous ammonia and subcutaneous strychnine for snakebite.

The diversities of specificity

What ultimately defeated *Serum Antivenimeux* in Australia was neither its preparation nor administration, but direct antagonism. Beyond his lucrative association with Gunn, Smith also demonstrated physiology at Sydney University. He was initially paired with Almroth Wright, later Britain's doyen of vaccination whose fleeting interest in venoms only arose after his one-year sojourn in Australia.[43] Wright's successor as the university's demonstrator in physiology, Charles Martin, had taught himself chemistry as an adolescent, before earning his medical degree and pursuing physiological training in Germany (Figure 27).[44]

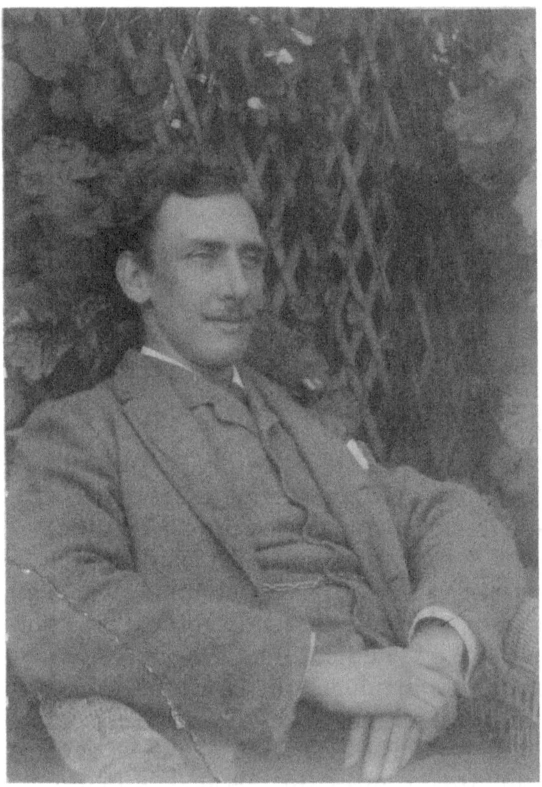

27 Charles James Martin, *c.*1892.

Immediately staking out venoms as primarily a chemical problem, Martin's lineage honoured neither Mueller nor Halford, but venom pharmacologists including Silas Weir Mitchell, Lucien Bonaparte and Alfred Wall. While it is perhaps unfair of Sharon Wallace to assert that Martin and Smith were 'the first Australian scientists to investigate venom and its action in an orderly, scientific fashion' (see Chapter 3), their mode of professionalised laboratory science proved a decisive schism.[45] They focused on black snake venom, believing it as potent as the cobra's. Thus demanding attention from investigators in India and Saigon, Martin iterated their tripartite task:

(1) What is the poison?
(2) What is its exact physiological action?
(3) How can one best prevent or counteract this action?[46]

While both snakes and humans remained remarkably absent from Martin's early publications, reagents and devices proliferated. His chemical mastery discerned in venom both a heat-labile proteid (albumen) and two temperature-refractory albumoses. Enlisting Board of Health bacteriologist Charles Pound to operate on guinea pigs, some had sponges infused with the poisonous proteids inserted subcutaneously; others suffered either whole or heat-treated venom injected into their jugular veins. These vivisections convinced Martin, Smith and Pound that albumoses embodied the toxic properties of both venom and 'the poisons produced by the bacilli of anthrax, diphtheria, and tubercle'.[47]

Creating remedies remained Martin's third priority. He possibly discussed neutralising serums with Smith, but by late 1892 the latter and Pound were investigating the air in Sydney's sewers, seemingly leaving *Serum Antivenimeux* to Calmette. Martin, moreover, set his sights on science – meaning to him the instrumented, reductionist pursuit of the fundamentals underlying physiological phenomena.[48] As Patricia Morison has delightfully painted, he was 'a gangling sensitive soul but a tough-minded scientist and a confirmed mechanist'.[49]

By 1893 he had 'arrived'. Martin's next paper appeared in the definitive *Journal of Physiology* – the first study involving Australian venoms ever to do so. Tellingly, his inquiry into coagulation disturbances effected by black snake venom was not prompted by clinical concerns. Rather, it followed an experimental observation: when dogs were cannulated to monitor their blood pressure after injecting venom, the tube did not become blocked with clotted blood. With Indian and European orthodoxy focusing on the paralytic – and hence neurological – actions of venom, Martin's paper echoed American interest in revealing 'highly important modifications in the constitution and character of the blood, under the influence of venom'.[50] These modifications, his vivisections and *in vitro* experiments revealed, were manifold. After envenoming frogs, dogs, cats and rabbits, Martin posited pronounced differences in susceptibility to the haematological effects of black snake venom – not just across species, but even between individual animals. Furthermore, repeated doses failed to replicate the initial effect: exposure apparently conferred a degree of immunity.

Arguing that blood was the seat of toxicity, Martin now claimed that Australian and Indian snake venoms were equipotent. Halford, verging on retirement, was delighted.[51] After two years systematically disaggregating black snake venom, on 3 July 1895 Martin presented his results to the Royal Society of New South Wales. This work was so comprehensive that it earned him the Society's Medal and a Doctorate of Science from London University.[52]

Boasting that his oeuvre 'was conducted entirely by experiments upon the lower animals', Martin derided observations from human cases as 'necessarily unsatisfactory owing to ignorance and want of control of so many factors'.[53] He voluntarily operated within British vivisection regulations, generally administering morphia – and occasionally ether or curare – to his instrumented, envenomed and monitored beasts. Nevertheless, Martin's colonial circumstances permitted him considerable latitude at a time when – as Michael Finn and James Stark argue – vivisection regulations forced regional British investigators to pursue non-interventional lines of inquiry.[54]

Technical innovation was foregrounded: a 'drip' for slowly infusing venom, an aërotonometer for ascertaining blood gases. Indeed, Martin's laboratory animals were essentially apparatus, connected in series to other instruments – a manometer to measure blood pressure, a smoked-drum kymograph to record respiratory amplitude. These inscription devices, more than the creatures' behaviour, determined his comprehension of venom as a physiological poison. It was precisely this disconnect between animals and their natural environment – one shared with humans – which British antivivisectionists insisted would undercut scientific claims to biological generality, notes Jed Mayer.[55] Martin considered canines poor experimental subjects precisely because their innate variations in size, basal physiology and responses to venom made replication of results problematic. In short, they were individuals. Yet Martin's papers indicated no consideration of their moral or sentimental worth – not even the hint of a wagging tail.

Likewise, Martin's elaborate apparatus broke venom down into a series of actions, requiring complex interventions and tracings to isolate their discrete physiological impact. Overall, he argued, black snake venom was an extraordinarily potent amalgam of toxins, superseded only by cobra venom and diphtheria toxine.[56] '*Pseudechis* venom is comprehensive in its action', Martin marvelled. 'It affects principally the three most vulnerable points in a higher organism; the blood, the heart, and the respiratory centre in the medulla.'[57]

The key differentiators were haematological: when rapidly introduced into the bloodstream, black snake venom caused massive intravascular coagulation; thereafter, the blood refused to clot. Conversely, slow infusions obviated the initial 'positive' clotting phase, so that only the 'negative' anticoagulant effect was observed. The fall in blood pressure unerringly revealed by his kymograph traces, Martin believed, was indicative of a direct cardiotoxic effect. Paralysis was likewise localised: that the vasomotor and vagus centres escaped toxicity, whilst the allied respiratory centre was profoundly retarded, comprised 'one of the most remarkable instances of the selective action of a poison, with which I am acquainted'.[58]

Martin's concurrent interest in the monotremes as rudimentary mammals fostered a collaboration with his eventual replacement, Frank Tidswell. Addressing the Linnean Society in July 1894, they foregrounded the 'remarkable analogy between the venom of Australian snakes and the poison of the Platypus'.[59] If these physiological data linking their poison to serpents did not lead to the demonisation of platypuses, it reinforced their denigration as 'primitive' mammals.[60]

As Martin's interest in venoms and toxins evolved, he devised diverse apparatuses to disaggregate these fluids. In particular, his high-pressure filter, which separated large molecules from solution onto a membrane of gelatin or silicic acid on clay, simplified the isolation of proteids.[61] Useful as this device proved analytically, it also acted analogically. His vivisections indicated that both toxicological and temporal disparities distinguished intravenous from subcutaneous administration of venom. Suggesting that black snake venom contained at least two toxins with differing levels of capillary permeability, Martin was convinced that these differences explained a significant proportion of both clinical and experimental variability following envenomation. While intravenous injection simultaneously distributed both fractions throughout the body, the paralytic effects of the more diffusible smaller molecule predominated upon subcutaneous administration.[62]

Circuiting his argument from principles to venoms, then back again, in 1897 Martin considered two serums entering clinical use: diphtheria antitoxin and Calmette's *antivenin*. Because both contained a putative antitoxic molecule likely to be a proteid, he argued, intravenous injection would greatly accelerate their curative effect.[63] Venoms thus provided his entrée to the wider world of immunological theory and praxis. As Martin wrote to a colleague in 1898: 'I am back working every day at diphtheria, snake-poison & their antitoxins.'[64]

The specificity paradox: killing universal antivenene, 1896–1904

Nothing brought Martin more international attention than the collision between his atomisation of Australian venoms and Calmette's 'universal' *antivenin*. Moving to Melbourne University in 1896 as its new physiology lecturer, Martin comprehensively usurped Halford as a teacher, an administrator and a scientist.[65] His promotion coincided with the arrival in Australia of an early batch of *Serum Antivenimeux*, following positive reports from the subcontinent the previous year.

This development, argues Chakrabarti, 'marginalised the British engagement with Indian snakes and venoms in colonial India'.[66] In Australia, however, its impact was nugatory. Making perhaps his final pronouncement as an experimenter, Halford declared that two bottles of *Serum Antivenimeux* he investigated were inert.[67] In February 1897, contemporaneous studies were conducted at the Board of Health Laboratories in Sydney and upon a pair of dogs at Melbourne Veterinary Hospital, overseen by representatives of the Victorian Central Board of Health and Calmette's Australian agents.[68] Both beasts died, yet the instructions accompanying *Serum Antivenimeux* not only cited animal testing to verify its potency, but outlined that when treating oxen, sheep, horses or dogs, it should be 'used in such cases just as in man, and in the same doses'.[69] Sales remained poor. By July the French Consulate-General offered 'any recognised medical or scientific institution … supplies of the serum free of charge for experimental purposes'.[70]

The horse, however, had bolted. Australian vivisections effectively poisoned *Serum Antivenimeux* before a single human case was attempted. In August 1897, Martin attacked both root and branch of Calmette's claims for a universal snakebite curative. Calmette – following Metchnikoff – believed that resistance to toxins lay within the tissues, and hence was subject to broad activation by antitoxins. Australian advocates of Behring's schema, including Martin, argued that a molecular relationship governed the highly specific affinity of circulating antitoxins for their toxin. As he pontificated, 'some actions of different kinds of snake venom are quite as distinct as, say, the actions of the toxins of tetanus and yellow fever'.[71]

Having generated the first Australian antivenene early in 1897 – a moderately effective serum against black snake venom – Martin now evaluated *Serum Antivenimeux* in rabbits and a few dogs. His black and tiger snake samples included whole venom and the diffusible, neurotoxic fraction which resembled 'in physiological action the preponderating constituent of cobra poison, if not indeed identical with it'. Mildly effective against this fraction, Martin concluded that overall, *Serum Antivenimeux* was 'practically useless as a remedial agent'.[72] Consequently, asserted the *Intercolonial Medical Journal of Australasia*, 'so far as Australia is concerned, we cannot regard Calmette's serum as a valuable remedy for the present'.[73]

Calmette retorted by attempting to isolate Australians – and Australian snakes. Aware that competition from Smith and Gunn's anthrax vaccine was hastening the demise of the Pasteur Institute of Australia, he was irked by the popularity of Mueller's 'universal' strychnine remedy. *Serum Antivenimeux* was proven worldwide, he asserted; being 'very often used for man and domestic animals (dogs, horses, oxen) ... none of those who have received the injection of serum, even after great delay, have succumbed to the effect of the snake poison'. Justifying centralised French manufacture, he argued that a single toxic property united all venoms globally: 'Everything depends in the resistance peculiar to the kind and size of the [envenomed] animal.'[74]

Promulgating his chemical metaphor, Martin argued that species was irrelevant; what counted was stoichiometry.[75] Collaborating with Thomas Cherry – later Melbourne University's first bacteriology lecturer – he combined diphtheria toxin or a tiger snake venom fraction with their respective antitoxins. Whether filtered or heated to inactivate the antitoxin, the resultant fluid proved inert in guinea pigs or rabbits. Reproducing these reactions *in vitro* – hence obviating exposure to bodily tissues – Martin and Cherry undermined Calmette and Metchnikoff's corporeal concept of antitoxin action, asserting that 'antagonism between the toxins of diphtheria and snake venom and their relative antitoxin is due to a direct chemical action'.[76] With debate escalating to the British medical periodicals, Martin drove home his point that these experimental lessons were applicable not just to snakebite, but the general principles underlying toxin–antitoxin interactions. As he boasted, 'it settles the point neatly & effectively'.[77]

On this note, Martin largely concluded his prolific Australian venom oeuvre. Elected a Fellow of the Royal Society in 1901 for original work on the chemistry and physiology of venoms, toxins and antitoxins, he moved to London in September 1903 as Director of the Lister Institute of Preventive Medicine. His Parthian shot was a lecture entitled 'Snakes and snake poison', in which he asserted that while tiger snake venom was the deadliest worldwide, the expense and specificity of antivenene dismissed it as a practical solution to Australia's snakebite problem.[78]

By 1897 the practitioner-hypothesiser era had effectively passed. Disaggregating Australian snake venoms via chemical and vivisectional data, Martin embodied the new experimental medicine. He was not alone: as venom historian Barbara Hawgood notes, over 1895–97 Vital Brazil differentiated the effects of two Brazilian snake venoms via vivisection. Subsequently inoculating dogs and goats to manufacture antivenenes, his 1898 trials corroborated Martin and dismissed Calmette: serums against one venom rarely counteracted others. By December 1901 the Brazilian Institute of Serumtherapy was manufacturing its own polyvalent antivenene.[79] Similar conclusions were soon reached in North America: having generated rattlesnake antiserum, in 1904 Hideyo Noguchi wrote to Mitchell that 'I am convinced of the falsehood of the bold claims made by Calmette.'[80] Concurrent British–Indian collaborations further demolished Calmette's universalism.[81]

Martin and Calmette, nevertheless, led the application of venom studies to reigning problems in immunity and immunotherapy. When in 1897 they jointly authored the venoms chapter for respected British textbook, *A System of Medicine*, Martin remarked, 'There is no toxine of which the details of the physiological action are so well known as those of some varieties of snake poison.'[82] By World War I, his stoichiometric model was effectively immunological orthodoxy.[83] Equally, claims Hawgood, 'Calmette's demonstration of anticobra serotherapy revolutionized the treatment of snakebite in man and domestic animals worldwide.'[84]

Paradoxically, in trumping Calmette, Martin stymied Australian research into snakebites until the late 1920s. His vivisections demonstrated the variety of venom components and their finely differentiated pathophysiological actions, but offered few diagnostic clues for doctors, let alone victims. Martin's black snake antivenene was never commercialised, and the only reported clinical use of *Serum Antivenimeux* in Australia occurred on 26 November 1900. Bitten by an unknown snake, a Victorian woman underwent ligature, suction, scarification and the inevitable brandy before Calmette's serum was injected. Although the attending doctor considered it 'a remedy worthy of more trial', sales collapsed thereafter.[85]

Transformation to instrumentation: the ambiguous impact of laboratory science

What remained, however, was Martin's approach to science – particularly vivisection. In June 1898 Tidswell (Figure 28) commenced injecting a horse with tiger snake venom. Following a painstakingly

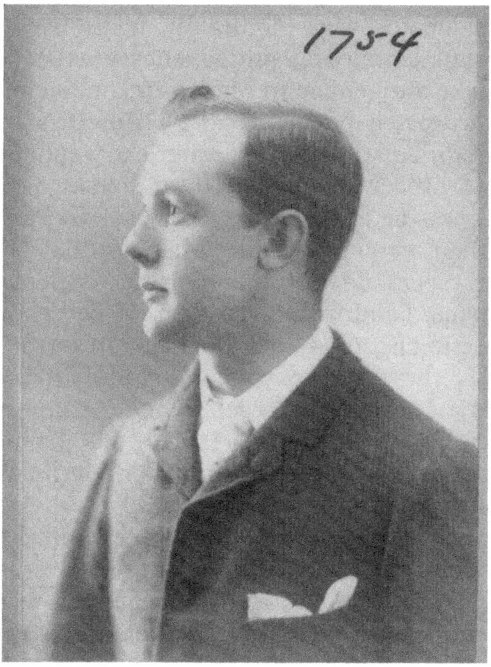

28 Frank Tidswell, 1892.

slow inoculation programme, by 1902 this equine could reportedly withstand a venom dose equivalent to that expressed by 22 tiger snakes – now deemed Australia's most dangerous serpent. Overall, Tidswell enumerated, 'the total amount received by the horse during the treatment (10 grammes) is about equal to the amount which would be yielded by 333 average snakes'.[86] The latter phrase was telling: after a highly instrumented milking procedure, both venom and serum were processed and homogenised – like milk – to blend out biological idiosyncrasies. Contemporaneous problems with inter-equine variability, notes Daniel Gilfoyle, led South African researchers to prioritise mules in early immunological research for horsesickness.[87]

Both the efficacy and specificity of Tidswell's tiger snake antivenene were confirmed by pitting it against lethal doses of venom. Indeed, his tests in rabbits suggested that tiger snake venom was even more potent than Martin had ventured. Noting drily that 'the serum obtained could validly be regarded as an antidote for tiger-snake venom', Tidswell found its efficacy enhanced when injected immediately and intravenously.[88] His *coup de grâce* comprised demonstrating that rabbits were not saved by *Serum Antivenimeux*, even at doses a thousandfold greater than the specific Australian product.[89]

If Australian snakes were nominally neutralised, circulation of their venoms and competing antivenenes escalated. Tidswell forwarded tiger snake antivenene to Martin in London and George Lamb in Bombay, who tested both this and Calmette's serum against a plethora of Indian, Australian and American venoms.[90] This Indian Medical Service officer inoculated local horses against cobra and daboia venoms, passing these antivenenes back to Tidswell for testing against Australian venoms. While Martin used Tidswell's serum to examine the specificity of the clotting ferment in Indian and Australian venoms, Lamb employed tiger snake venom to differentiate the haemolytic effects of snake poisons *in vitro*.[91] Indeed, noted Tidswell in 1906, 'the present day view is entirely to the effect that the toxic principles are different in each venom', comprising 'independent toxic principles – hæmolysins, leucolysins, hæmorrhagins, neurolysins, agglutinins, fibrin ferments, antifibrin ferments, neurotoxins, cardiotoxins, antibacteriolysins, &c.'[92]

Venoms thereby became autonomous biochemical tools. The final pre-war Australian venom studies – those of Sydney University physiologists David Welsh and Henry Chapman – barely mentioned snakes.[93] By 1914, international investigators freely traded Australian venoms, employing them largely to investigate blood biochemistry and physiology.[94]

Paradoxically, this global exchange only enhanced parochialism. In debunking universal antidotes, venom investigators emphasised both the particularity of indigenous serpents and the necessity for local scientific solutions. Yet if Tidswell's antivenene was generated 'for the elucidation of the question of specificity', he seemed almost jubilant that its clinical effectiveness was so tightly constrained. Because each venom required a separate antivenene, he concluded baldly in 1906, 'snake-bite would appear to be for the moment beyond the sphere of practical serotherapy'.[95]

His message stuck. That year Ernest Black, President of Western Australia's Central Board of Health, advised that 'Dr Tidswell ... has prepared a reliable antivenin serum but I am not aware that it is procurable. The only other successful treatment is the hypodermic injection of strychnine.'[96] As serum therapy for infectious diseases marched triumphantly forward, antivenenes became a byway. Acknowledging its theoretical advantages, popular authors concurred that as a cure, antivenene was 'almost useless'.[97] In almost the last Australian venom paper published before 1914, Welsh and Chapman asserted that 'treatment by antivenin (or polyvalent antivenins) can never supersede the rational and scientific local treatment of the wound'.[98]

What, then, were Australians left with? While Mueller's strychnine therapy persisted into the 1950s, the final 'scientific' remedy for snakebite proved decidedly lowbrow. As the *Chemist and Druggist of Australasia* declared in 1907, 'The permanganate of potash remedy for snake bite is now the only one that any trust can be put in.'[99] Brunton, Joseph Fayrer and Indian Medical Service physician Leonard Rogers had together announced this 'new' agent in 1904. The eminent trio's triumph was not the chemical – well known as Condy's crystals and widely employed by doctors, pharmacists and laity – but its container. Their pocket-sized device included a blade for scarifying the bite site and a recess containing crystals to pour onto the venom, allegedly neutralising it *in situ*. It hardly heralded medical modernity in the manner of Halford's syringe in 1870, or Calmette's and Fraser's antivenenes in 1895. Although Rogers demonstrated its efficacy via a series of vivisections in Britain, ironically this culmination of four decades of Indian snakebite research required human cases to garner clinical acceptance.[100] By 1914 the best medical advice for snakebitten Australians literally just scratched the surface.

Vestiges

Thus a half-century of seeking a 'specific' against snake venom collapsed in the face of growing biomedical insistence on specificity. What remained was prosaic first aid. In 1898 Australian Museum zoologist Edgar Waite produced the first new monograph on local ophidians since 1869. Medical men and chemists should 'make a special point of knowing the hurtful snakes', he suggested, because 'the remedies applied may be, in themselves, a source of danger' (Figure 29).[101] Yet Waite said nothing of how he knew which snakes were dangerous; unlike his predecessor Gerard Krefft, Waite was no vivisector.

Agreeing with Waite that there were but five potentially deadly Australian serpents, in 1906 Tidswell faced some awkward facts. Analysing snakebite reports from medical periodicals, the Government Statistician and police returns submitted across New South Wales since 1891, he identified only four likely 'killers': the death adder plus tiger, black and brown snakes. The 'superb snake' or copperhead – central to Underwood's 1850s demonstrations – remained lethal by reputation only. Embarrassingly, given his and Martin's strenuous characterisation of its venom, Tidswell admitted that no human death occurred among 87 black snake bites. His list shrank to three. He furthermore concluded that the only treatment improving outcome after snakebite was ligature, reducing case mortality rates from 55.5% to 25.4%.[102]

Long of interest to police, Boards of Health and Departments of Public Instruction, by Federation of the Australian colonies in 1901,

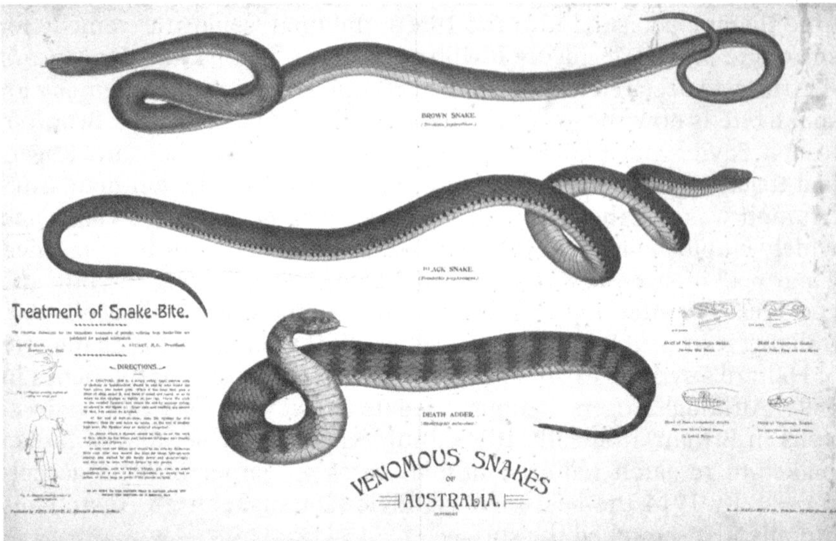

29 Thomas Shine, *Venomous Snakes of Australia* (Sydney: W.M. Maclardy & Co., 1895).

snakebite seemed a government responsibility. After 1906, Tidswell crafted a new facility, state funded but – he hoped – operating semi-autonomously to extend beyond public health into diseases of veterinary and agricultural import. Charles Pound fostered similar ambitions for Brisbane's Queensland Stock Institute.[103] Tidswell's New South Wales Bureau of Microbiology (1909–13), argues Peter Tyler, was modelled on both the Pasteur and Lister Institutes – the latter headed by Martin.[104] If the 1900 bubonic plague outbreak in Sydney interrupted Tidswell's antivenene programme, it also highlighted the dearth of local serum facilities, leading to limited vaccine manufacture by his Bureau.

Antivenene production, however, was never attempted. Serums, contemporaries lamented, were expensive to manufacture and required temperature-regulated storage. While vaccine matter was relatively stable, by 1902 Tidswell knew of Lamb's studies in India showing that *Serum Antivenimeux* rapidly deteriorated in hot localities.[105] Its very logistics required state succour and control, from electrification to macadamisation. Yet a comparison with smallpox vaccination questions why government subsidies were not forthcoming. Rebekah McWhirter tables 107 deaths from smallpox in Australia from 1852 to 1903.[106] Similarly incomplete and unreliable sources suggest at least 414 deaths attributed to snakebite over 1864–1926, including 119 in 1882–92 alone. But, as McWhirter adds, 'the contemporary attitude towards smallpox was that it was undesirable, it could and should be avoided, and – crucially – it was the state's duty to achieve that end'.[107]

'The involvement of the state from the outset', remarks Mazumdar of early serological therapy, 'meant that by the side of the technical process of standardization, lay the political.'[108] Australian circumstances proved no exception. Scientists working within serum facilities – like Tidswell and Pound – harnessed calls from primary industry to agitate for state centralisation and subsidisation of research and technology. Medically, as Claire Hooker and Alison Bashford have shown, after 1890 epidemiology and bacteriology intersected with governmentality as states – and especially the new Australian Commonwealth – aspired to control population health via diphtheria immunisation and serum therapy.[109] Critically, however, non-indigenous pathogens such as anthrax and diphtheria were both ontologically discrete and globally homogeneous.

The fundamental problem inhibiting Australian production of the purportedly 'universal' technology of antivenenes lay in the diversity of snakes. Successes were subject to the vagaries of 'nature' – the rare and unpredictable event of snakebite, correct identification of serpents, clinical evaluation of severity and the unique biochemical complexity of each species' venom. The characteristics and behaviour of the animals themselves largely negated any medicinal benefits of antivenene, fatally compromising cost:benefit ratios.

In pre-war Australia, as chemists, bureaucrats and scientists acknowledged, this was a step too far. It took World War I – and the abnegation of German patents, mobilisation of local chemical manufacture and importation of serum production expertise – to craft a robust local therapeutics industry. In 1925, one of the first research projects posited by the new Commonwealth Serum Laboratories was a series of antivenenes.[110] Tiger snake antivenene was first marketed in 1930 while the next product – a veterinary antitoxin for tick paralysis – emerged in 1938.[111] Domesticated animals, as always, remained intricately associated with the epistemology and technology of neutralising indigenous venoms.

Reproving his Indian critics and their vile vivisections, in 1895 Augustus Mueller paraphrased Gratiano in *The Merchant of Venice*: 'When I speak let no dog bark.'[112] The irony was twofold. Henceforth, scientific medicine – at least as applied to venoms and antidotes – could never again reside merely in clinical testimony. Vivisection, the experimental employment of animals to create and verify new knowledge, was now the established pathway to epistemological sovereignty. The second irony was that in laboratories, dogs no longer barked. Once autonomous actors, like the snakes that bit them, they were now silenced technological artefacts. Whether their tails drooped or wagged became irrelevant; only isolated tracings, tabulated numbers and microscopic observations 'spoke' to vivisectors.

For snakes, the dismemberments of the laboratory proved doubly disfiguring. Drained of their poison, serpents faded from consideration. It was now their venom – autonomous, active and above all specific – that became the primary unit of analysis. Yet as venom was in turn atomised into discrete fractions, scientific medicine was defeated precisely by this diversity and complexity. In this sense, snakes never conceded their integrity, nor their natural sovereignty.

Notes

1 See for example Christopher Lawrence, *Medicine in the Making of Modern Britain, 1700–1920* (London: Routledge, 1994), pp. 71–6; W.F. Bynum, 'The rise of science in medicine, 1850–1913', in W.F. Bynum *et al.* (eds), *The Western Medical Tradition, 1800 to 2000* (Cambridge: Cambridge University Press, 2006), pp. 111–13.

2 Jonathan Simon, 'Monitoring the stable at the Pasteur Institute', *Science in Context*, 21:2 (2008), p. 196; see also Axel C. Hüntelmann, 'Evaluation as a practical technique of administration: the regulation and standardization of diphtheria serum', in Christoph Gradmann and Jonathan Simon (eds), *Evaluating and Standardizing Therapeutic Agents, 1890–1950* (Basingstoke: Palgrave Macmillan, 2010), pp. 31–51.

3 Ilana Löwy, 'On guinea pigs, dogs and men: anaphylaxis and the study of biological individuality, 1902–1939', *Studies in History and Philosophy of Biological and Biomedical Sciences*, 34:3 (2003), pp. 399–423; Michael E. Lynch, 'Sacrifice and the transformation of the animal body into a scientific object: laboratory culture and ritual practice in the neurosciences', *Social Studies of Science*, 18:2 (1988), pp. 265–89.

4 Pratik Chakrabarti, 'Beasts of burden: animals and laboratory research in colonial India', *History of Science*, 48:2 (2010), p. 137; see also E.M. Tansey, 'The Wellcome Physiological Research Laboratories 1894–1904: the Home Office, pharmaceutical firms, and animal experiments', *Medical History*, 33:1 (1989), pp. 1–41.

5 See Claire Hooker, 'Sanitary failure and risk: pasteurisation, immunisation and the logics of prevention', in Alison Bashford and Claire Hooker (eds), *Contagion: Epidemics, History and Culture from Smallpox to Anthrax* (Annandale: Pluto Press, 2002), pp. 135–43.

6 T.P. Anderson Stuart, 'Anniversary address', *Journal and Proceedings of the Royal Society of New South Wales*, 28 (1894), p. 12.

7 G.B. Halford, *Thoughts, Observations, and Experiments on the Action of Snake Venom on the Blood. With an Appendix* (Melbourne: Stillwell and Co., 1894), p. 69.

8 John V. Pickstone and Michael Worboys, 'Introduction', *Isis*, 102:1 (2011), p. 99.

9 Henry Sewall, 'Experiments on the preventive inoculation of rattlesnake venom', *Journal of Physiology*, 8:3–4 (1887), p. 204.

10 T. Lauder Brunton, 'Remarks on snake venom and its antidotes', *British Medical Journal*, 1:1566 (1891), pp. 2–3.

11 Pratik Chakrabarti, *Bacteriology in British India: Laboratory Medicine and the Tropics* (Rochester: University of Rochester Press, 2012), p. 140.

12 Arthur M. Silverstein, *A History of Immunology* (San Diego: Academic Press, 1989), pp. 38–54, 88–93; Alfred I. Tauber and Leon Chernyak, *Metchnikoff and the Origins of Immunology: from Metaphor to Theory* (New York: Oxford University Press, 1991), pp. 101–53.

13 Pauline M.H. Mazumdar, *Species and Specificity: An Interpretation of the History of Immunology* (Cambridge: Cambridge University Press, 1995), pp. 8–9.
14 See Alan Cribb, Joan Cribb, and John Pearn, 'Pituri, plants and physic', in John Pearn and Lawrie Powell (eds), *The Bancroft Tradition* (Brisbane: Amphion Press, 1991), pp. 73–4; I.M. Mackerras and Elizabeth N. Marks, 'The Bancrofts: a century of scientific endeavour', *Proceedings of the Royal Society of Queensland*, 84:1 (1973), pp. 12–13.
15 T.L. Bancroft, 'Strychnine, a useless remedy in snake-bite', *Proceedings of the Royal Society of Queensland*, 8:2 (1891), p. 81.
16 Thos. L. Bancroft, 'On the scrub tick', *Queenslander* (3 January 1891), p. 36.
17 Thos. L. Bancroft, 'Some further observations on the physiological action of snake venom, together with a reference to the strychnine cure of snakebite', *Australasian Medical Gazette*, 13 (1894), pp. 228–9.
18 Thos. L. Bancroft, 'On snakebite', *Australasian Medical Gazette*, 12 (1893), p. 44.
19 Thomas R. Fraser, 'On the rendering of animals immune against the venom of the cobra and other serpents; and on the antidotal properties of the blood-serum of the immunized animals', *Proceedings of the Royal Society of Edinburgh*, 20 (1895), p. 452.
20 *Ibid.*, p. 451. It may well have been a mulga snake, *Pseudechis australis* (Ken Winkel and Jeanette Covacevich, personal communications).
21 *Ibid.*, p. 456.
22 Thomas R. Fraser, 'Further observations on antivenene, and on the production of immunity against serpents' venom; with an account of the antidotal properties of the blood serum of venomous serpents', *Proceedings of the Royal Society of Edinburgh*, 20 (1895), pp. 473–4.
23 Thomas R. Fraser, 'On the rendering of animals immune against the venom of the cobra and other serpents', p. 459. Italics in original.
24 T.R. Fraser, 'An address on immunization against serpents' venom, and the treatment of snake-bite with antivenene', *British Medical Journal*, 1:1842 (1896), p. 960.
25 See especially Annick Guénel, 'The creation of the first overseas Pasteur Institute, or the beginning of Albert Calmette's Pastorian career', *Medical History*, 43:1 (1999), pp. 5–8, 14–16; Barbara J. Hawgood, 'Doctor Albert Calmette 1863–1933: founder of antivenomous serotherapy and of antituberculous BCG vaccination', *Toxicon*, 37:9 (1999), p. 1244.
26 A. Calmette, 'Contribution a l'étude du venin des serpents. Immunisation des animaux et traitement de l'envenimation', *Annales de l'Institut Pasteur*, 8:5 (1894), pp. 280–8.
27 *Ibid.*, p. 276n; A. Calmette, 'Propriétés du sérum des animaux immunisés contre les venins de diverses espèces de serpents', *Comptes Rendus Hebdomadaires des Séances de l'Académie des Sciences*, 118:18 (1894), pp. 1004–5.
28 Halford, *Thoughts, Observations, and Experiments on the Action of Snake Venom on the Blood*, p. 69.
29 Guénel, 'The creation of the first overseas Pasteur Institute', pp. 16–17.
30 A. Calmette, 'The treatment of animals poisoned with snake venom by the injection of antivenomous serum', *British Medical Journal*, 2:1859 (1896), pp. 399–400.
31 J.S. Chaussivert, 'Letters regarding the "Pasteur Mission" in Australia', in Jean Chaussivert and Maurice Blackman (eds), *Louis Pasteur and the Pasteur Institute in Australia* (Kensington: University of New South Wales, 1988), p. 21.
32 Rebekah McWhirter, '"Lymph or liberty": responses to smallpox vaccination in the eastern Australian colonies' (PhD thesis, University of Tasmania, 2008), pp. 41–7; Alison S. Day, 'Child immunisation: reactions and responses to New Zealand government policy 1920–1990' (PhD thesis, University of Auckland, 2008), pp. 27–8; David Evans, 'Vaccine lymph: some difficulties with logistics in colonial Victoria, 1854–1874', in John Pearn and Catherine O'Carrigan (eds), *Australia's Quest for Colonial Health: Some Influences on Early Health and Medicine in Australia* (Brisbane: Department of Child Health, Royal Children's Hospital, 1983), pp. 160–1, 172–5, 177n1.

33 Alison Bashford, 'Foreign bodies: vaccination, contagion and colonialism in the nineteenth century', in Alison Bashford and Claire Hooker (eds), *Contagion: Epidemics, History and Culture from Smallpox to Anthrax* (Annandale: Pluto Press, 2002), pp. 42–6, 52–4.

34 Phyllis M. Rountree, 'The Pasteur Institute and Australia', in Jean Chaussivert and Maurice Blackman (eds), *Louis Pasteur and the Pasteur Institute in Australia* (Kensington: University of New South Wales, 1988), pp. 9–12; Stephen Dando-Collins, *Pasteur's Gambit: Louis Pasteur, the Australasian Rabbit Plague and a Ten Million Dollar Prize* (North Sydney: Vintage, 2008), pp. 178–84.

35 Ian Parsonson, *The Australian Ark: A History of Domesticated Animals in Australia* (Collingwood: CSIRO Publishing, 2000), pp. 233–8.

36 Jan Todd, 'The Pasteur Institute of Australia – success and failure', in Jean Chaussivert and Maurice Blackman (eds), *Louis Pasteur and the Pasteur Institute in Australia* (Kensington: University of New South Wales, 1988), pp. 25–34. This conclusion is somewhat disputed by James F. Stark, 'Anthrax and Australia in a global context: the international exchange of theories and practices with Britain and France, c.1850–1920', *Health & History*, 14:2 (2012), pp. 10–14, 18–19.

37 New South Wales, *An Act to Provide Against the Communication of Infectious Diseases to Animals*, 51 Vict. 30 (16 March 1888), section 3.

38 Jan Todd, *Colonial Technology: Science and the Transfer of Innovation to Australia* (Cambridge: Cambridge University Press, 2009), pp. 93–5.

39 Dr. Katz, 'Notes and exhibits', *Proceedings of the Linnean Society of New South Wales*, 3 (second series) (1888), p. 401.

40 Claire Hooker and Alison Bashford, 'Diphtheria and Australian public health: bacteriology and its complex applications, c. 1890–1930', *Medical History*, 46:1 (2002), pp. 46–53.

41 Bashford, 'Foreign bodies', pp. 39–45.

42 See Paul Weindling, 'From medical research to clinical practice: serum therapy for diphtheria in the 1890s', in John V. Pickstone (ed.), *Medical Innovations in Historical Perspective* (New York: St Martin's Press, 1992), pp. 74–80; Cay-Rüdiger Prüll, 'Paul Ehrlich's standardization of serum: Wertbestimmung and its meaning for twentieth-century biomedicine', in Christoph Gradmann and Jonathan Simon (eds), *Evaluating and Standardizing Therapeutic Agents, 1890–1950* (Basingstoke: Palgrave Macmillan, 2010), pp. 16–19.

43 Michael Worboys, 'Vaccine therapy and laboratory medicine in Edwardian Britain', in John V. Pickstone (ed.), *Medical Innovations in Historical Perspective* (New York: St Martin's Press, 1992), pp. 87–102.

44 See especially Harriette Chick, 'Charles James Martin. 1866–1955', *Biographical Memoirs of Fellows of the Royal Society*, 2 (1956), pp. 173–5; Martin Gibbs, *Charles Martin: His Life and Letters* (London: Martin Gibbs, 2011), pp. 10–20.

45 Sharon Louise Wallace, 'Treatment of snakebite from Halford to Sutherland' (BMedSci thesis, University of Melbourne, 1983), p. 81.

46 C.J. Martin and J.McG. Smith, 'The venom of the Australian black snake, (*Pseudechis porphyriacus*)', *Journal and Proceedings of the Royal Society of New South Wales*, 26 (1892), p. 240.

47 *Ibid.*, p. 262.

48 Muriel Robertson and Keith Inglis, 'Charles James Martin. 9th January 1866–15th February 1955', *Journal of Pathology and Bacteriology*, 71:2 (1956), p. 523.

49 Patricia Morison, *JT Wilson and the Fraternity of Duckmaloi* (Amsterdam: Editions Rodopi, 1997), p. 92.

50 C.J. Martin, 'On some effects upon the blood produced by the injection of the venom of the Australian black snake (*Pseudechis porphyriacus*)', *Journal of Physiology*, 15:4 (1893), p. 400.

51 University of Melbourne Archives, Melbourne, 1981.0062, Halford, George Britton, 'Letters responding to appeal for snakes heads – Aug–Sept 1894', Charles Martin to George Halford, 13 September 1894.

52 Barbara J. Hawgood, 'Sir Charles James Martin MB FRS: Australian serpents and Indian plague, one-hundred years ago', *Toxicon*, 35 (1997), pp. 1001–4.
53 C.J. Martin, 'On the physiological action of the venom of the Australian black snake (*Pseudechis porphyriacus*)', *Journal and Proceedings of the Royal Society of New South Wales*, 29 (1895), p. 147.
54 Michael A. Finn, and James F. Stark, 'Medical science and the Cruelty to Animals Act 1876: a re-examination of anti-vivisectionism in provincial Britain', *Studies in History and Philosophy of Science Part C: Studies in History and Philosophy of Biological and Biomedical Sciences*, 49 (2015), pp. 20–2.
55 Jed Mayer, 'The nature of the experimental animal: evolution, vivisection, and the Victorian environment', in Carol Freeman, Elizabeth Leane and Yvette Watt (eds), *Considering Animals: Contemporary Studies in Human–Animal Relations* (Farnham: Ashgate, 2011), pp. 98–103.
56 *Ibid.*, pp. 151–2, 157.
57 *Ibid.*, p. 274.
58 *Ibid.*, p. 218.
59 C.J. Martin and Frank Tidswell, 'Observations on the femoral gland of *Ornithorhynchus* and its secretion; together with an experimental enquiry concerning its supposed toxic action', *Proceedings of the Linnean Society of New South Wales*, 9 (second series) (1895), p. 497.
60 Peter Hobbins, 'A spur to atavism: placing platypus poison', *Journal of the History of Biology*, 48:4 (2015), pp. 521–2.
61 C.J. Martin, 'A rapid method of separating colloids from crystalloids in solutions containing both', *Journal of Physiology*, 20:4–5 (1896), pp. 367–9.
62 C.J. Martin, 'An explanation of the marked difference in the effects produced by subcutaneous and intravenous injection of the venom of Australian snakes', *Journal and Proceedings of the Royal Society of New South Wales*, 30 (1897), pp. 150–1, 156–7.
63 C.J. Martin, 'On the advisability of administering curative serum by intravenous injection', *Intercolonial Medical Journal of Australasia*, 2 (1897), pp. 537–8.
64 University of Sydney Archives, Sydney (hereafter UoSA), P162, J.T. Wilson family archives, 1895–1933, Charles Martin to James Wilson, 23 February 1898, p. 1.
65 R.J.W. Selleck, *The Shop: The University of Melbourne 1850–1939* (Carlton: Melbourne University Press, 2003), pp. 392–4; Juliet Flesch, *Life's Logic: 150 Years of Physiology at the University of Melbourne* (North Melbourne: Australian Scholarly Publishing, 2012), pp. 16–20.
66 Chakrabarti, *Bacteriology in British India*, p. 113.
67 'Treatment of snakebite', *Australasian Journal of Pharmacy*, 12 (1897), p. 5.
68 'Snakebite and antidote', *Queenslander* (20 February 1897), pp. 420–1; Frank Tidswell, 'A preliminary note on the serum-therapy of snake-bite', *Australasian Medical Gazette*, 21 (1902), pp. 177–8.
69 'Anti-venomous serum or "antivenene". Instructions for use of', *South Australian Government Gazette*, 2 (1897), p. 1329.
70 'Calmette's serum for snake-bite', *Chemist and Druggist of Australasia*, 12:6 (1897), p. 141.
71 C.J. Martin, 'The curative value of Calmette's anti-venomous serum in the treatment of inoculations with the poisons of Australian snakes', *Intercolonial Medical Journal of Australasia*, 2 (1897), p. 528.
72 *Ibid.*, pp. 531–2.
73 'Snake-bite', *Intercolonial Medical Journal of Australasia*, 2 (1897), p. 553.
74 A. Calmette, 'On the curative value of the "antivenomous serum" in relation to the poisons of Australian and Indian snakes', *Intercolonial Medical Journal of Australasia*, 3 (1898), pp. 193, 196.
75 C.J. Martin, 'The curative value of Calmette's anti-venomous serum in the treatment of inoculations with the poisons of Australian snakes (a rejoinder to M. Le Dr. Calmette)', *Intercolonial Medical Journal of Australasia*, 3 (1898), p. 201.

76 C.J. Martin and T. Cherry, 'The nature of the antagonism between toxins and antitoxins', *Proceedings of the Royal Society of London*, 63:400 (1898), p. 426.
77 UoSA P162 3 Item 3, Charles Martin to James Wilson, 8 July 1898, p. 2. See also C.J. Martin, 'Further observations concerning the relation of the toxin and anti-toxin of snake-venom', *Proceedings of the Royal Society of London*, 64:403 (1899), p. 89.
78 'Snake poisoning and its antidotes', *Chemist and Druggist of Australasia*, 19:2 (1904), p. 50.
79 Barbara J. Hawgood, 'Pioneers of anti-venomous serotherapy: Dr Vital Brazil (1865–1950)', *Toxicon*, 30:5–6 (1992), pp. 575–6.
80 Hideyo Noguchi, 'Immunization against rattlesnake venom (communicated by S. Weir Mitchell)', *Transactions of the Association of American Physicians*, 19 (1904), p. 48.
81 For example R.H. Elliot, W.C. Sillar and George S. Carmichael, 'On the action of the venom of *Bungarus cœruleus* (the common krait)', *Proceedings of the Royal Society of London*, 74 (1904), p. 109; Thomas R. Fraser and R.H. Elliot, 'Contributions to the study of the action of sea-snake venoms. – Part I. Venoms of *Enhydrina valakadien* and *Enhydris curtus*', *Philosophical Transactions of the Royal Society of London. Series B, Containing Papers of a Biological Character*, 196 (1905), pp. 259–60.
82 C.J. Martin and A. Calmette, 'Snake-poison and snake-bite', in Thomas Clifford Allbutt (ed.), *A System of Medicine*, 2 (London: MacMillan, 1897), p. 834.
83 For instance, Hans Zinsser, *Infection and Resistance: An Exposition of the Biological Phenomena Underlying the Occurrence of Infection and the Recovery of the Animal Body from Infectious Disease* (New York: The Macmillan Company, 1914), pp. 104–7, 464–6.
84 Hawgood, 'Doctor Albert Calmette', p. 1249.
85 G. Bill, 'Notes on a case of snake-bite, treated with antivenine', *Intercolonial Medical Journal of Australasia*, 7 (1902), p. 348.
86 Frank Tidswell, 'A preliminary note on the serum-therapy of snake-bite', *Veterinarian*, 75 (1902), p. 178.
87 Daniel Gilfoyle, 'Veterinary immunology as colonial science: method and quantification in the investigation of horsesickness in South Africa, c. 1905–1945', *Journal of the History of Medicine and Allied Sciences*, 61:1 (2006), pp. 38–41.
88 Frank Tidswell, *Researches on Australian Venoms. Snake-Bite, Snake-Venom and Antivenine. The Poison of the Platypus. The Poison of the Red-Spotted Spider* (Sydney: William Applegate Gullick, 1906), p. 56.
89 Frank Tidswell, 'A preliminary note on the serum-therapy of snake-bite', p. 180. I therefore disagree with Peter Mirtschin, 'The pioneers of venom production for Australian antivenoms', *Toxicon*, 48:7 (2006), pp. 900–1.
90 G. Lamb, *Specificity of Antivenomous Sera* (Calcutta: Office of the Superintendent of Government Printing, India, 1903), pp. 4–6, 10–13.
91 George Lamb, *Snake-venoms in Relation to Haemolysis* (Calcutta: Office of the Superintendent of Government Printing, India, 1905), pp. 3–5.
92 Tidswell, *Researches on Australian Venoms*, p. 30.
93 D.A. Welsh and H.G. Chapman, 'Concerning snake venom', *Australasian Medical Gazette*, 29 (1910), pp. 348–9.
94 For instance, John Mellanby, 'The coagulation of the blood. Part 2. The action of snake venoms, peptone and leech extract', *Journal of Physiology*, 38:6 (1909), pp. 444–76; Mlle Newtonoff, 'Le venin du Pseudechis porphyriacus d'Australie (black-snake)' (MD thesis, Université de Lausanne, 1912), p. 16; Mlle Starorypinska, 'Immunisation contre l'action coagulante du venin de Pseudechis porphyriacus' (MD thesis, Université de Lausanne, 1913), p. 16.
95 Tidswell, *Researches on Australian Venoms*, pp. 35, 37.
96 State Records Office of Western Australia, Perth, 1907/0459 Consignment 1003, Snake bites – re cure for, Ernest Black to WJ Rae, 21 February 1906.
97 Donald MacDonald, *The Bush Boy's Book*, 2nd edn (Sydney: Cornstalk Publishing, 1927), p. 277.

98 Welsh and Chapman, 'Concerning snake venom', p. 345.
99 'Snake bite remedies', *Chemist and Druggist of Australasia*, 22:7 (1907), p. 182.
100 Leonard Rogers, *Happy Toil: Fifty-five Years of Tropical Medicine* (London: Frederick Muller, 1950), pp. 97–100; Lauder Brunton, Joseph Fayrer and Leonard Rogers, 'Experiments on a method of preventing death from snake bite, capable of common and easy practical application', *Proceedings of the Royal Society of London*, 73 (1904), p. 323.
101 Edgar R. Waite, *A Popular Account of Australian Snakes With a Complete List of the Species and an Introduction to Their Habits and Organisation* (Sydney: Thomas Shine, 1898), p. 23.
102 Tidswell, *Researches on Australian Venoms*, pp. 5, 16–21.
103 Beverley Margaret Angus, *Tick Fever and the Cattle Tick in Australia 1829–1996* (Palm Beach: BM Angus, 2003), pp. 21–4, 38–42, 55–8.
104 Peter J. Tyler, 'Our first microbiologist', *Locality* (2001), p. 12.
105 G. Lamb and Wm. Hanna, *Standardisation of Calmette's Anti-Venomous Serum with Pure Cobra Venom: The Deterioration of This Serum through Keeping in India* (Calcutta: Office of the Superintendent of Government Printing, India, 1902), p. 11.
106 McWhirter, 'Lymph or Liberty', p. 28. She acknowledges that her sources are incomplete and almost certainly an underestimate.
107 *Ibid.*, p. 49.
108 Pauline M.H. Mazumdar, 'The state, the serum institutes and the League of Nations', in Christoph Gradmann and Jonathan Simon (eds), *Evaluating and Standardizing Therapeutic Agents, 1890–1950* (Basingstoke: Palgrave Macmillan, 2010), p. 118.
109 Hooker and Bashford, 'Diphtheria and Australian Public Health'.
110 A.H. Brogan, *Committed to Saving Lives: A History of the Commonwealth Serum Laboratories* (South Yarra: Hyland House, 1990), pp. 1–4, 43–4.
111 Peter G. Hobbins, 'Serpentine science: Charles Kellaway and the fluctuating fortunes of venom research in interwar Australia', *Historical Records of Australian Science*, 21:1 (2010), pp. 10–11.
112 A. Mueller, 'Discoursive notes on snake poison and the strychnine treatment', *Indian Medical Record*, 8 (1895), p. 209.

CONCLUSION

Published in 1906, Frank Tidswell's *Researches on Australian Venoms* effectively bookended the colonial era of venom research in Australia. Few of the topics, statistics or therapeutics he explored were meaningfully revisited until 1927.[1] His title was telling. Animals were absent: Tidswell examined *venoms*. That they were *Australian* was critical: potent and complex agents, venoms were also indigenous and autonomous. What, however, of *researches*?

This book has argued that vivisection – interventional studies conducted in animals, with the intent of generating knowledge – was central to how snakes and their toxins were known in colonial Australia. Rather than authoritative pronouncements issued by isolated investigators, snakebite experiments were marked by crowd participation and plebeian expertise. Indeed, it was largely popular demand which drove antipodean doctors and naturalists to adopt vivisection, at a time when Britons were apathetic – if not actively antipathetic – to this methodology. Under negotiation was not merely the outcome of animal experimentation, but its very epistemology. Into the 1880s, public snakebite displays and audiences dictated what counted as proof, including the necessary conditions, performances and practitioners. If not democratic, such knowledge remained insistently demotic.

My mission has been to rewrite beasts back into consideration, both as sentient beings and as integral participants in the emergent structures of colonial science. White settlers came to know venomous snakes primarily through their interactions with domestic animals. This association operated within a wider colonial animal matrix that governed commercial, sentimental and ethical hierarchies and equivalences between beasts. If not unique, Australia proved an outlier in co-colonisation by European humans and animals. Indigenous fauna were so alien, and familiar beasts so valuable, that the metonymy linking non-human and human invaders held tightly. From patent antidotes to injected antisera, snakebitten animals comprised both experimental subjects and potential patients for remedies legitimated via vivisection.

Snakes themselves remained exceptional. Resisting white dominion in a way that few other indigenous vertebrates could, they fostered opprobrium by association, lessening ethical consideration for all animals used in snakebite experiments. Paradoxically, their exceptionalism was highlighted by the conjoint growth of Australian nativism and pointedly 'amateur' natural history. After 1880 a new wave of field naturalist groups embraced the simple pleasures of nature study introduced via classrooms, zoological gardens, museums and Arcadian columns in daily newspapers. Each urged encountering 'Nature' experientially, yet such idylls were all too often shattered when meandering naturalists encountered a snake and gave chase with shotgun or sapling.[2] Indeed, one of the earliest and loudest voices amongst the new nativists belonged to James Barrett, the first man to hold conjoint Vivisection Licenses in Britain and Victoria.[3]

What field naturalists rejected was a growing atomisation. Throughout the preceding century, as a 1903 primary-school textbook bewailed, 'the single robe of Nature was torn into separate parts called Sciences, which seemed to have no connection; and a jumble of facts was presented, under the name of Natural History'.[4] In 1895 the first text devoted to Australian zoology was dominated by serpents on account – its author explained – of insistent 'inquiries in parliament, in the press, and in other places, for information on the poisonous snakes so dangerous to human life'.[5] Zoologists remained devoted to descriptive minutiae, biogeography and anecdotes to characterise Australian ophidians, yet at a more fundamental level, serpents eluded nascent ideas of ecology and evolution. How their venom arose, why it was so biochemically complex, what roles it served, and whether it hallmarked progress or atavism, largely went unasked.

The historical ontology of venom is a second stream coursing through this book. From dragon's breath to 'germinal matter', it traced a remarkable journey from 1600 to 1900. If in 1788 an animal's malevolence passed into its poison, by 1888 attributions flowed largely in the reverse direction. Perhaps the most remarkable trope was the regular conflation of animal venoms with infectious matter, from syphilis to diphtheria. This association is rarely remarked in the rich historiography of disease, yet from the Renaissance to the *fin de siècle*, venom served as the exemplar for discrete, exogenous agents of illness. The shared descriptor 'virus' is particularly intriguing in the nineteenth-century context, suggesting a foreign interloper capable of not just perturbing, but to some extent subverting the victim's animal economy. Existential concern over such contamination was surprisingly absent in nineteenth-century accounts of envenomation. Nevertheless, the ontology of venom as contagion – or as an autonomous entity – promises rich territory for posthumanist scholarship addressing the insistent question of 'the animal'.

One refrain developed early in my research was that wherever I sought snakes I found dogs, and wherever I captured dogs I detected police. This triad suggests numerous avenues for further inquiry, from legal histories of animal violence and control, through to emotional reconstructions of pet-keeping and sentimentality in settler society. Conversely, in this book Aboriginal voices have been almost entirely refracted through scientific sources. As the nuanced scholarship of Pratik Chakrabarti suggests, non-Eurocentric perspectives can constructively rescript the historiographies of tropical medicine, dangerous beasts and Imperial governance.[6] An entirely different history of Indigenous ways of knowing and responding to venomous animals, both pre- and post-contact, awaits attention by enthnobiologists, zooarchaeologists, historical anthropologists and Indigenous historians.

Venomous encounters has outlined layers of popular investment in the pursuit of pragmatic knowledge, especially as embodied in variants of 'scientific medicine'. Vivisectional studies of venomous snakes typified the ebb and flow of information and investigative practice between laity and often self-appointed cognoscenti. Participation in such active experimentation suggests a need to rework histories which paint colonials as profuse collectors of information, but omit their role in generating and circulating 'useful knowledge'. Concurrently, the mundanity of colonial vivisection provides a striking contrast with

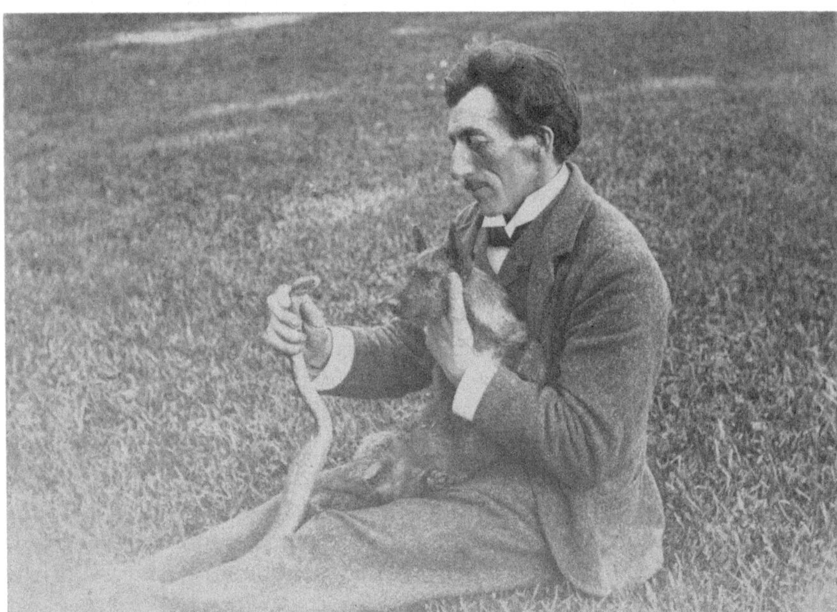

30 Dudley Le Souef, 'Davis', 1895.

the protracted public and parliamentary debates on its morality in Victorian Britain. Was this truly the same Empire?

The voices of animals remain largely silent throughout this history. Their tribulations rarely troubled contemporaries who observed the sacrifice of pets in pubs (Figure 30). This is not to suggest that Britons were literally brutalised by the particularities of colonial circumstance. Rather, settler society pragmatics commoditised animals: the welfare of individual beasts carried little economic or moral weight. The resultant profligacy with animal life, especially for indigenous species and 'vermin', bothered few commentators.

The years after World War I heralded a new world. If the serpent-slaying kookaburra was now revered as a national icon, snakes – and the spasmodic Australian obsession with snakebite – receded even further from the happenstance of everyday life. Snakes themselves continued adapting to their new environments, but as agents they slithered further down the animal matrix. Quarantined from nativist protection, drained of their venom and neutralised by a parade of putative remedies, they stared unblinkingly back.

Notes

1 See Peter G. Hobbins, 'Serpentine science: Charles Kellaway and the fluctuating fortunes of venom research in interwar Australia', *Historical Records of Australian Science*, 21:1 (2010), pp. 1–34.

2 Examples abound, but see for instance D. Best, 'A holiday excursion to North Mirboo', *Victorian Naturalist*, 6 (1890), p. 82. See furthermore Tom Griffiths, '"The natural history of Melbourne": the culture of nature writing in Victoria, 1880–1945', *Australian Historical Studies*, 23:93 (1989), pp. 344–50; John Cleland, 'Reminiscences of the early days of the Field Naturalists' Section of the Royal Society of S.A.', *South Australian Naturalist*, 44:2 (1969), pp. 21–2.

3 James Barrett, 'General introduction', in James W. Barrett (ed.), *Save Australia: A Plea for the Right Use of Our Flora and Fauna* (Melbourne: Macmillan & Co., 1925), pp. 1–15.

4 William Gillies and Robert Hall, *Nature Studies in Australia, with a Natural History Calendar, Summaries of the Chapters, and Complete Index* (Melbourne: Whitcombe & Tombs, 1903), p. iii.

5 G. Metcalfe, *Australian Zoology* (Sydney: E.W. Cole, 1895), p. v. In contrast, see T. Jeffery Parker and William A. Haswell, *A Text-book of Zoology*, 2 (London: Macmillan and Co., 1897), p. 340.

6 Pratik Chakrabarti, *Bacteriology in British India: Laboratory Medicine and the Tropics* (Rochester: University of Rochester Press, 2012), pp. 113–41.

BIBLIOGRAPHY

Archives

Archives Office of Tasmania (Hobart)
Minutes, annual reports and press reports of the Southern Branch of the RSPCA

National Library of Australia (Canberra)
Manuscripts

Public Records Office of Victoria (Melbourne)
Chief Secretary's Office

State Library of New South Wales (Sydney)
Mitchell Library

State Library of Victoria (Melbourne)
La Trobe collection

State Records Office of Western Australia (Perth)
Chief Secretary's Office

University of Melbourne (Melbourne)
Ann Tovell Archives
University of Melbourne Archives

University of Sydney (Sydney)
University of Sydney Archives

Newspapers and periodicals

Age (Melbourne)
Agricultural Gazette of New South Wales
Annales de l'Institut Pasteur
Annals and Magazine of Natural History
Argus (Melbourne)
Asiatick Researches
Australasian (Melbourne)
Australasian Journal of Pharmacy
Australasian Medical Gazette
Australasian Nurses Journal
Australasian Sketcher with Pen and Pencil (Melbourne)

Australian Magazine (Sydney)
Australian Medical Gazette
Australian Medical Journal
British Medical Journal
Bulletin Général de Thérapeutique Médicale et Chirurgicale
California Medical Gazette
Chemist and Druggist of Australasia
Comptes Rendus Hebdomadaires des Séances de l'Académie des Sciences
Edinburgh Medical Journal
Examiner (Launceston)
Hamilton Spectator
Hobart Town Gazette and Southern Reporter
Illustrated Australian News for Home Readers (Melbourne)
Illustrated Sydney News
Indian Medical Gazette
Indian Medical Record
Intercolonial Medical Journal of Australasia
Journal and Proceedings of the Royal Society of New South Wales
Journal of Physiology
Journal of the Transactions of the Victoria Institute, or Philosophical Society of Great Britain
Lancet
Medical and Surgical Reporter
Medical & Surgical Review (Australasian)
Medical Record of Australia
Medical Times and Gazette
Melbourne Medical Record
New South Wales Medical Gazette
New York Medical Journal
North American Medico-chirurgical Review
Papers and Proceedings of the Royal Society of Tasmania
Papers and Proceedings of the Royal Society of Van Diemen's Land
Philosophical Transactions: Giving Some Account of the Present Undertakings, Studies and Labours of the Ingenious in Many Considerable Parts of the World
Philosophical Transactions of the Royal Society of London. Series B, Containing Papers of a Biological Character
Proceedings of the Linnean Society of New South Wales
Proceedings of the Royal Society of Edinburgh
Proceedings of the Royal Society of London
Proceedings of the Royal Society of Queensland
Proceedings of the Royal Society of Victoria
Proceedings of the Zoological Society of London
Queanbeyan Age and General Advertiser
Queenslander (Brisbane)
Speculum

Sydney Gazette and New South Wales Advertiser
Sydney Magazine of Science and Art
Tasmanian Journal of Natural Science, Agriculture, Statistics, &c
Therapeutic Gazette
Transactions and Proceedings of the Royal Society of Victoria
Transactions of a Society for the Improvement of Medical and Chirurgical Knowledge
Transactions of the Association of American Physicians
Veterinarian
Victorian Naturalist
Virchows Archiv für Pathologische Anatomie und Physiologie und für Klinische Medizin

Official sources

Cardwell, Edward, Lord Winmarleigh, E.W. Forster, J.B. Karslake, T.H. Huxley, John Eric Erichsen, Richard Holt Hutton and Nathaniel Baker, *Report of the Royal Commission on the Practice of Subjecting Live Animals to Experiments for Scientific Purposes; with Minutes of Evidence and Appendix*. Vol. C.1397 and C.1397-I (London: Her Majesty's Stationery Office, 1876).
Cleland, J.B., 'Alleged snake-bite remedies', in *Report of the Director-General of Public Health New South Wales, for the Year Ended 31st December, 1913* (Sydney: Government Printer, 1915), p. 250.
Ewart, Joseph, Vincent Richards, and S. Coull Mackenzie, *Report on the Effects of Artificial Respiration, Intravenous Injection of Ammonia and Administration of Various Drugs, &c., in Indian and Australian Snake-Poisoning; and the Physiological, Chemical, and Microscopical Nature of Snake Poisons. By the Commission Appointed to Investigate the Subject* (Calcutta: Bengal Secretariat Press, 1874).
New South Wales, *An Act to Provide Against the Communication of Infectious Diseases to Animals*, 51 Vict. 30, 16 March 1888.
South Australian Government Gazette.
United Kingdom, *An Act to Amend the Law Relating to Cruelty to Animals*, 39 & 40 Vict. c. 77, 15 August 1876.
Victoria, *An Act for the Protection of Animals*, 45 Vict. 712, 24 December 1881.
Victoria. *Parliamentary Debates. Session 1881. Legislative Council and Legislative Assembly* (Melbourne: John Ferres, 1882).
Victoria Government Gazette.

Unpublished theses

Buckley, R.L., 'Six dogs: a saga of snakes, dogs and medical byways' (BA (Hons) thesis, La Trobe University, 2003).
Day, Alison S., 'Child immunisation: reactions and responses to New Zealand government policy 1920–1990' (PhD thesis, University of Auckland, 2008).

Drayson, Nick, 'Early developments in the literature of Australian natural history: together with a select bibliography of Australian natural history writing, printed in English, from 1697 to the present' (PhD thesis, Australian Defence Force Academy, University of New South Wales, 1997).

Haynes, Elsie Frances, 'Edward Swarbreck Hall: medical scientist and social reformer in colonial Tasmania' (MA thesis, University of Tasmania, 1976).

Hoffman, Daniel John, 'Fatal attractions: curare-based arrow poisons, from medical innovation to lethal injection' (PhD thesis, University of California, 2009).

MacCulloch, Jennifer, 'Creatures of culture: the animal protection and preservation movements in Sydney, 1880–1930' (PhD thesis, University of Sydney, 1993).

McWhirter, Rebekah, '"Lymph or liberty": responses to smallpox vaccination in the eastern Australian colonies' (PhD thesis, University of Tasmania, 2008).

Newtonoff, Mlle, 'Le venin du Pseudechis porphyriacus d'Australie (black-snake)' (MD thesis, Université de Lausanne, 1912).

Slouber, Michael James, 'Gāruda medicine: a history of snakebite and religious healing in South Asia' (PhD thesis, University of California, 2012).

Starorypinska, Mlle, 'Immunisation contre l'action coagulante du venin de Pseudechis porphyriacus' (MD thesis, Université de Lausanne, 1913).

Wallace, Sharon Louise, 'Treatment of snakebite from Halford to Sutherland' (BMedSci thesis, University of Melbourne, 1983).

Published sources

A.R., *True and Wonderfull a Discourse Relating to a Strange and Monstrous Serpent (or Dragon) Lately Discouered* (London: Iohn Trundle, 1614).

An Emigrant Mechanic, *Settlers and Convicts: or Recollections of Sixteen Years' Labour in the Australian Backwoods* (Carlton: Melbourne University Press, 1969).

An Old Bushman, *Bush Wanderings of a Naturalist; or, Notes on the Field Sports and Fauna of Australia Felix* (London: Routledge, Warne, & Routledge, 1861).

Anderson, Kay, 'A walk on the wild side: a critical geography of domestication', *Progress in Human Geography*, 21:4 (1997), 463–85.

Anderson, Kay, 'Culture and nature at the Adelaide Zoo: at the frontiers of "human" geography', *Transactions of the Institute of British Geographers*, 20:3 (1995), 275–94.

Anderson, Virginia DeJohn, *Creatures of Empire: How Domestic Animals Transformed Early America* (Oxford: Oxford University Press, 2004).

Anderson, Warwick, *The Collectors of Lost Souls: Turning Kuru Scientists into Whitemen* (Baltimore: Johns Hopkins University Press, 2008).

Angus, Beverley Margaret, *Tick Fever and the Cattle Tick in Australia 1829–1996* (Palm Beach: BM Angus, 2003).

Apjohn, James, 'Toxicology', in John Forbes, Alexander Tweedie and John Conolly (eds), *The Cyclopædia of Practical Medicine*, vol. 4 (London: Sherwood, Gilbert, and Piper, and Baldwin and Cradock, 1835), pp. 189–243.

Appadurai, Arjun, 'Introduction: commodities and the politics of value', in Arjun Appadurai (ed.), *The Social Life of Things: Commodities in Cultural Perspective* (Cambridge: Cambridge University Press, 1986), pp. 3–63.

Arnold, David, 'The politics of poison: healing, empowerment and subversion in nineteenth-century India', in David Hardiman and Projit Bihari Mukharji (eds), *Medical Marginality in South Asia: Situating Subaltern Therapeutics* (Abingdon: Routledge, 2012), pp. 171–92.

Attewell, Guy, 'Interweaving substance trajectories: tiryaq, circulation and therapeutic transformation in the nineteenth century', in Anne Digby, Waltraud Ernst and Projit B. Mukharji (eds), *Crossing Colonial Historiographies: Histories of Colonial and Indigenous Medicines in Transnational Perspective* (Newcastle upon Tyne: Cambridge Scholars Publishing, 2010), pp. 1–20.

Australian Museum, *A Catalogue of the Specimens of Natural History and Miscellaneous Curiosities Deposited in the Australian Museum* (Sydney: James Tegg, 1837).

Baer, George M., 'The history of rabies', in Alan C. Jackson and William H. Wunner (eds), *Rabies*, 2nd edn (Amsterdam: Elsevier, 2007), pp. 1–22.

Baker, Henry, *The Microscope Made Easy*, 5th edn (London: J. Dodsley, 1769).

Baker, K.D., 'Vivisection debate in nineteenth century Great Britain: a muted echo in colonial and early post-colonial Australia', *Australian Veterinary Journal*, 76:10 (1998), 683–9.

Baldwin, Martha, 'The snakestone experiments: an early modern medical debate', *Isis*, 86:3 (1995), 394–418.

Ball, C., 'Joseph Clover and the cobra: a tale of snake envenomation and attempted resuscitation with bellows in London, 1852', *Anaesthesia and Intensive Care*, 38:1 (2010), 5–9.

Barrett, James, *Eighty Eventful Years* (Melbourne: J.C. Stephens, 1945).

Barrett, James, 'General introduction', in James W. Barrett (ed.), *Save Australia: A Plea for the Right Use of Our Flora and Fauna* (Melbourne: Macmillan & Co., 1925), pp. 1–15.

Barrow, Mark V. Jr, 'The alligator's allure: changing perceptions of a charismatic carnivore', in Dorothee Brantz (ed.), *Beastly Natures: Animals, Humans, and the Study of History* (Charlottesville: University of Virginia Press, 2010), pp. 127–53.

Basalla, George, 'The spread of Western science', *Science*, 156:3775 (1967), 611–22.

Bashford, Alison, 'Foreign bodies: vaccination, contagion and colonialism in the nineteenth century', in Alison Bashford and Claire Hooker (eds), *Contagion: Epidemics, History and Culture from Smallpox to Anthrax* (Annandale: Pluto Press, 2002), pp. 39–60.

Beauties of Natural History; Or, Elements of Zoography (London: Richardson and Urquhart, 1777).

Bennett, Tony, *Anthropological Assemblages: Producing Culture as a Surface of Government* (Milton Keynes: Centre for Research on Socio-Cultural Change, 2008).

Berncastle, Dr, *Australian Snake Bites: Their Treatment and Cure. The Use and Abuse of Tobacco* (Melbourne: Mason Firth & Co., 1868).

Bertomeu-Sánchez, José Ramón, 'Popularizing controversial science: a popular treatise on poisons by Mateu Orfila (1818)', *Medical History*, 53:3 (2009), 351–78.

Birke, Lynda, *Feminism, Animals and Science: The Naming of the Shrew* (Buckingham: Open University Press, 1994).

Blainey, Geoffrey, *A Centenary History of the University of Melbourne* (Melbourne: Melbourne University Press, 1957).

Boddice, Rob, 'Vivisecting Major: a Victorian gentleman scientist defends animal experimentation, 1876–1885', *Isis*, 102:2 (2011), 215–37.

Bowler, Richard, 'Broadmarsh, Tasmania', in Eric Rolls (ed.), *Visions of Australia: Impressions of the Landscape 1642–1910* (South Melbourne: Thomas C. Lothian, 2002), pp. 125–6.

Boyce, James, 'A dog's breakfast ... lunch and dinner: canine dependency in early Van Diemen's Land', *Tasmanian Historical Research Association Papers and Proceedings*, 51:4 (2004), 194–213.

Boyce, James, *Van Diemen's Land* (Melbourne: Black, 2008).

Brasier, Angeline, 'Prisoners' bodies: methods and advances in convict medicine in the transportation era', *Health and History*, 12:2 (2010), 18–38.

Bresalier, Michael, 'Neutralizing flu: "immunological devices" and the making of a virus disease', in Kenton Kroker, Jennifer Keelan and Pauline M.H. Mazumdar (eds), *Crafting Immunity: Working Histories of Clinical Immunology* (Aldershot: Ashgate, 2008), pp. 108–44.

Brogan, A.H., *Committed to Saving Lives: A History of the Commonwealth Serum Laboratories* (South Yarra: Hyland House, 1990).

Brookes, R., *The General Practice of Physic*, 5th edn, vol. 2 (London: J. Newbery, 1765).

Brown, Karen, *Mad Dogs and Meerkats: A History of Resurgent Rabies in Southern Africa* (Cape Town: University of Cape Town Press, 2011).

Bryan, Benjamin (ed). *The Vivisectors' Directory: Being a List of the Licensed Vivisectors in the United Kingdom, Together with the Leading Physiologists in Foreign Laboratories* (London: Victoria Street Society for the Protection of Animals from Vivisection, United with the International Association for the Total Suppression of Vivisection, 1884).

Buckingham, John, *Bitter Nemesis: The Intimate History of Strychnine* (Boca Raton: CRC Press, 2008).

Budd, Wallace B., *Hear the Other Side: The R.S.P.C.A. in South Australia, 1875–1988* (Hawthorndene: Investigator Press, 1988).

Buettinger, Craig, 'Women and antivivisection in late nineteenth-century America', *Journal of Social History*, 30:4 (1997), 857–72.

Buffon, Georges Louis Leclerc, *Natural History: General and Particular*, vol. 2 (Edinburgh: William Creech, 1780).

Buffon, Georges Louis Leclerc, *Natural History of Birds, Fish, Insects and Reptiles* (London: J.S. Barr, 1793).

Burnett, D. Graham, *Trying Leviathan: The Nineteenth-Century New York Court Case that Put the Whale on Trial and Challenged the Order of Nature* (Princeton: Princeton University Press, 2007).

Butcher, Barry W., 'Gorilla warfare in Melbourne: Halford, Huxley and "Man's place in nature"', in R.W. Home (ed.). *Australian Science in the Making* (Cambridge: Cambridge University Press, 1988), pp. 153–69.

Bynum, W.F., '"C'est un malade": animal models and concepts of human diseases', *Journal of the History of Medicine and Allied Sciences*, 45:3 (1990), 397–413.

Bynum, W.F., *Science and the Practice of Medicine in the Nineteenth Century* (Cambridge: Cambridge University Press, 1994).

Bynum, W.F., 'The rise of science in medicine, 1850–1913', in W.F. Bynum *et al.* (eds), *The Western Medical Tradition, 1800 to 2000* (Cambridge: Cambridge University Press, 2006), pp. 103–239.

Cambridge, Ada, '(Arriving in Melbourne)', in Elizabeth Webby (ed.), *Colonial Voices: Letters, Diaries, Journalism and Other Accounts of Nineteenth-Century Australia* (St Lucia: University of Queensland Press, 1989), pp. 43–7.

Campbell, C.H., 'Dr. Mueller's strychnine cure of snake-bite', *Medical Journal of Australia*, 2 (1968), 1–8.

Campbell, C.H., 'Professor Halford's germ theory of snake poisoning', *Medical Journal of Australia*, 1 (1966), 552–5.

Campbell, C.H., 'Professor Halford's new treatment of snake bite with the injection of ammonia into the veins', *Medical Journal of Australia*, 1 (1966), 1008–15.

Cann, John, *Historical Snakeys* (Rodeo: ECO Publishing, 2014).

Cann, John, *Snakes Alive! Snake Experts & Antidote Sellers of Australia* (Kenthurst: Kangaroo Press, 1986).

Cervetti, Nancy, 'S. Weir Mitchell and his snakes: unraveling the "united web and woof of popular and scientific beliefs"', *Journal of Medical Humanities*, 28:3 (2007), 119–33.

Chakrabarti, Pratik, *Bacteriology in British India: Laboratory Medicine and the Tropics* (Rochester: University of Rochester Press, 2012).

Chakrabarti, Pratik, 'Beasts of burden: animals and laboratory research in colonial India', *History of Science*, 48:2 (2010), 125–51.

Chakrabarti, Pratik, *Materials and Medicine: Trade, Conquest and Therapeutics in the Eighteenth Century* (Manchester: Manchester University Press, 2010).

Charas, Moyse, *New Experiments Upon Vipers Containing Also an Exact Description of All the Parts of a Viper, the Seat of Its Poyson, and the Several Effects Thereof* (London: J. Martyn, 1670).

Chaussivert, J.S., 'Letters regarding the "Pasteur Mission" in Australia', in Jean Chaussivert and Maurice Blackman (eds), *Louis Pasteur and the Pasteur Institute in Australia* (Kensington: University of New South Wales, 1988), pp. 17–24.

Chick, Harriette, 'Charles James Martin. 1866–1955', *Biographical Memoirs of Fellows of the Royal Society*, 2 (1956), 172–208.

Cleland, J.B., 'Aborigines: diseases and medicines', in *Australian Encyclopaedia*, 2nd edn, vol. 1 (Sydney: Angus & Robertson, 1958), pp. 82–7.

Cleland, John, 'Reminiscences of the early days of the Field Naturalists' Section of the Royal Society of S.A.', *South Australian Naturalist*, 44:2 (1969), 21–3.

Clode, Danielle, 'From molluscs to monkeys: Darwin and early Australian biology', in Jeanette Hoorn (ed.), *Reframing Darwin: Evolution and the Arts in Australia* (South Carlton: Melbourne University Press, 2009), pp. 62–79.

Cohen, Esther, 'Animals in medieval perceptions: the image of the ubiquitous other', in Aubrey Manning and James Serpell (eds), *Animals and Human Society: Changing Perspectives* (London: Routledge, 1994), pp. 59–80.

Coleman, William, *Biology in the Nineteenth Century: Problems of Form, Function, and Transformation* (Cambridge: Cambridge University Press, 1985).

Coleman, William, 'The cognitive basis of the discipline: Claude Bernard on physiology', *Isis*, 76:1 (1985), 49–70.

Collins, David, *An Account of the English Colony in New South Wales: With Remarks On the Dispositions, Customs, Manners, &c. of the Native Inhabitants of That Country*, vol. 1 (London: T. Cadell Jun. and W. Davies, 1798).

Connah, Graham, *The Archaeology of Australia's History* (Cambridge: Cambridge University Press, 1993).

Covacevich, Jeanette, 'Phangs and physic: 40,000 years of risky business', in John Pearn and Mervyn Cobcroft (eds), *Fevers and Frontiers* (Brisbane: Department of Child Health, University of Queensland, 1990), pp. 61–72.

Cowen, David L., and William H. Helfand, *Pharmacy: An Illustrated History* (New York: Harry N. Abrams, 1990).

Cribb, Alan, Joan Cribb and John Pearn, 'Pituri, plants and physic', in John Pearn and Lawrie Powell (eds), *The Bancroft Tradition* (Brisbane: Amphion Press, 1991), pp. 61–74.

Crosby, Alfred W., *Ecological Imperialism: The Biological Expansion of Europe, 900–1900* (Cambridge: Cambridge University Press, 1986).

Cross, Stephen J., 'John Hunter, the animal oeconomy, and late eighteenth-century physiological discourse', in William Coleman and Camille Limoges (eds), *Studies in History of Biology* (Baltimore: Johns Hopkins University Press, 1981), pp. 1–110.

Crowther, W.E.L.H., 'A case of so-called hydrophobia: a matter of diagnosis', *Medical Journal of Australia*, 1 (1946), 69–72.

Crowther, W.E.L.H., 'Mr. Charles Underwood and his antidote, with some observations on snake bite in Tasmania', *Medical Journal of Australia*, 1 (1956), 83–90.

Cunningham, D.D., 'Salts of strychnia as remedies for snake-bite', in Robert Bird (ed.), *Transactions of the First Indian Medical Congress held at St. Xavier's College, Calcutta, 24th to 29th December, 1894* (Calcutta: Caledonian Steam Printing Works, 1895), pp. 488–90.

Cunningham, Peter, *Two Years in New South Wales*, 2nd edn, vol. 1 (Sydney: Angus and Robertson in association with the Royal Australian Historical Society, 1966).

Cushing, Nancy, and Kevin Markwell, 'Platypus diplomacy: animal gifts in international relations', *Journal of Australian Studies*, 33:3 (2009), 255–71.

Dale, Leigh, 'Empire's proxy: sheep and the colonial environment', in Helen Tiffin (ed.), *Five Emus to the King of Siam: Environment and Empire* (Amsterdam: Rodopi, 2007), pp. 3–11.

Dando-Collins, Stephen, *Pasteur's Gambit: Louis Pasteur, the Australasian Rabbit Plague and a Ten Million Dollar Prize* (North Sydney: Vintage, 2008).

Daston, Lorraine, 'On scientific observation', *Isis*, 99:1 (2008), 97–110.

Daston, Lorraine, and Peter Galison, *Objectivity* (New York: Zone Books, 2007).

Daudin, F.M., *Histoire Naturelle, Générale et Particulière des Reptiles* (Paris: F. Dufart, 1803 [Année XI]).

Dawson, James, *Australian Aborigines: The Languages and Customs of Several Tribes of Aborigines in the Western District of Victoria, Australia* (Melbourne: George Robertson, 1881).

Degeling, Chris, 'Canines, consanguinity, and one-medicine: all the qualities of a dog except loyalty', *Health and History*, 10:2 (2008), 23–47.

Derrida, Jacques, 'The animal that therefore I am (more to follow)', trans. David Willis, *Critical Inquiry*, 28 (2002), 369–418.

Di Gregorio, Mario A., 'In search of the natural system: problems of zoological classification in Victorian Britain', *History and Philosophy of the Life Sciences*, 4 (1982), 227–54.

Drayton, Richard, 'Science, Medicine, and the British Empire', in Robin W. Winks and Alaine Low (eds), *The Oxford History of the British Empire* (Oxford: Oxford University Press, 1999), pp. 264–76.

Duke, J., 'The symptoms and treatment of snake bite in India with special mention of Dr. A. Mueller's subcutaneous injection of strychnine, based on the consideration of 37 cases', in Robert Bird (ed.), *Transactions of the First Indian Medical Congress Held at St. Xavier's College, Calcutta, 24th to 29th December, 1894* (Calcutta: Caledonian Steam Printing Works, 1895), pp. 490–8.

Dunlap, Thomas R., *Nature and the English Diaspora: Environment and History in the United States, Canada, Australia, and New Zealand* (Cambridge: Cambridge University Press, 1999).

Earles, M.P., 'The experimental investigation of viper venom by Felice Fontana (1730–1805)', *Annals of Science*, 16:4 (1960), 255–68.

Evans, David, 'Vaccine lymph: some difficulties with logistics in colonial Victoria, 1854–1874', in John Pearn and Catherine O'Carrigan (eds), *Australia's Quest for Colonial Health: Some Influences on Early Health and Medicine in Australia* (Brisbane: Department of Child Health, Royal Children's Hospital, 1983), pp. 157–82.

Evans, Raymond, '"Plenty shoot 'em": the destruction of Aboriginal societies along the Queensland frontier', in A. Dirk Moses (ed.), *Genocide and Settler*

Society: Frontier Violence and Stolen Indigenous Children in Australian History (New York: Berghahn Books, 2004), pp. 150–73.

Fabbri, Christiane Nockels, 'Treating medieval plague: the wonderful virtues of theriac', *Early Science and Medicine*, 12:3 (2007), 247–83.

Fayrer, Joseph, *Recollections of My Life* (Edinburgh: William Blackwood and Sons, 1900).

Fayrer, Joseph, *The Thanatophidia of India. Being a Description of the Venomous Snakes of the Indian Peninsula, With an Account of the Influence of Their Poison on Life and a Series of Experiments* (London: J. and A. Churchill, 1872).

Finch, Lynette, 'Soothing syrups and teething powders: regulating proprietary drugs in Australia, 1860–1910', *Medical History*, 43:1 (1999), 74–94.

Finn, Michael A., and James F. Stark, 'Medical science and the Cruelty to Animals Act 1876: a re-examination of anti-vivisectionism in provincial Britain', *Studies in History and Philosophy of Science Part C: Studies in History and Philosophy of Biological and Biomedical Sciences*, 49 (2015), 12–23.

Finney, Colin, *Paradise Revealed: Natural History in Nineteenth-Century Australia* (Melbourne: Museum of Victoria, 1993).

Fitzpatrick, Kathleen, *Sir John Franklin in Tasmania 1837–1843* (Melbourne: Melbourne University Press, 1949).

Flesch, Juliet, *Life's Logic: 150 Years of Physiology at the University of Melbourne* (North Melbourne: Australian Scholarly Publishing, 2012).

Flinders, Matthew, *Observations On the Coasts of Van Diemen's Land, On Bass's Strait and Its Islands, and On Part of the Coasts of New South Wales* (London: John Nichols, 1801).

Foley, Paul, '*Duboisia myoporoides*: the medical career of a native Australian plant', *Historical Records of Australian Science*, 17:1 (2006), 31–69.

Fontana, Felice, *Treatise On the Venom of the Viper; On the American Poisons; and On the Cherry Laurel, and Some Other Vegetable Poisons* (London: J. Murray, 1787).

Foucault, Michel, 'On the archaeology of the sciences: response to the Epistemology Circle', trans. Robert Hurley, in James D. Faubion (ed.), *Aesthetics: Essential Works of Foucault 1954–1984* (London: Penguin Books, 1998), pp. 297–333.

Frank, Robert G., 'The telltale heart: physiological instruments, graphic methods, and clinical hopes 1854–1914', in William Coleman and Frederic L. Holmes (eds), *The Investigative Enterprise: Experimental Physiology in Nineteenth-Century Medicine* (Berkeley: University of California Press, 1988), pp. 211–90.

Franklin, Adrian, *Animal Nation: The True Story of Animals and Australia* (Sydney: University of New South Wales Press, 2006).

Franklin, Adrian, *Animals and Modern Cultures: A Sociology of Human–Animal Relations in Modernity* (London: Sage, 1999).

Freeman, Carol, *Paper Tiger: A Visual History of the Thylacine* (Leiden: Brill, 2010).

French, Richard D., *Antivivisection and Medical Science in Victorian Society* (Princeton: Princeton University Press, 1975).

Fudge, Erica, *Perceiving Animals: Humans and Beasts in Early Modern English Culture* (Urbana: University of Illinois Press, 2002).

Fye, W. Bruce, 'S. Weir Mitchell, Philadelphia's "lost" physiologist', *Bulletin of the History of Medicine*, 57 (1983), 188–202.

Gandevia, Bryan, and Ann Tovell, 'The first Australian medical libraries', *Medical Journal of Australia*, 2 (1964), 314–20.

Garrison, Fielding H., *An Introduction to the History of Medicine, with Medical Chronology, Suggestions for Study and Bibliographic Data*, 2nd edn (Philadelphia: W.B. Saunders and Company, 1917).

Gibbs, Martin, *Charles Martin: His Life and Letters* (London: Martin Gibbs, 2011).

Gilfoyle, Daniel, 'Veterinary immunology as colonial science: method and quantification in the investigation of horsesickness in South Africa, c. 1905–1945', *Journal of the History of Medicine and Allied Sciences*, 61:1 (2006), 26–65.

Gilfoyle, Daniel, 'Veterinary research and the African rinderpest epizootic: the Cape Colony, 1896–1898', *Journal of Southern African Studies*, 29:1 (2003), 133–54.

Gillies, William, and Robert Hall, *Nature Studies in Australia, with a Natural History Calendar, Summaries of the Chapters, and Complete Index* (Melbourne: Whitcombe & Tombs, 1903).

Goldsmith, Oliver, *An History of the Earth, and Animated Nature*, 2nd edn, vol. 7 (London: J. Nourse, 1779).

Goodrick, Joan, *Life in Old Van Diemens Land* (London: Robert Hale, 1978).

Gossel, Patricia Peck, 'William Henry Welch and the antivivisection legislation in the District of Columbia, 1896–1900', *Journal of the History of Medicine and Allied Sciences*, 40:4 (1985), 397–419.

Govett, William Romaine, *Sketches of New South Wales* (Melbourne: Gaston Renard, 1977).

Gradmann, Christoph, 'Locating therapeutic vaccines in nineteenth-century history', *Science in Context*, 21:2 (2008), 145–60.

Griffin, J.P., 'Venetian treacle and the foundation of medicines regulation', *British Journal of Clinical Pharmacology*, 58:3 (2004), 317–25.

Griffiths, Tom, '"The natural history of Melbourne": the culture of nature writing in Victoria, 1880–1945', *Australian Historical Studies*, 23:93 (1989), 339–65.

Guénel, Annick, 'The creation of the first overseas Pasteur Institute, or the beginning of Albert Calmette's Pastorian career', *Medical History*, 43:1 (1999), 1–25.

Guerrini, Anita, *Experimenting with Humans and Animals: From Galen to Animal Rights* (Baltimore: Johns Hopkins University Press, 2003).

Gunther, Albert E., *A Century of Zoology at the British Museum through the Lives of Two Keepers, 1815–1914* (London: Dawsons, 1975).

Günther, Albert C.L.G., *The Reptiles of British India* (London: Robert Hardwicke, 1864).

Hacking, Ian, 'Do we see through a microscope?' *Pacific Philosophical Quarterly*, 62 (1981), 305–22.

Hacking, Ian, *Historical Ontology* (Cambridge, Mass.: Harvard University Press, 2002), pp. 1–26.

Haines, Gregory, *Pharmacy in Australia: The National Experience* (North Sydney: Australian Pharmaceutical Publishing Company, 1988).

Halford, G.B., *Thoughts, Observations, and Experiments on the Action of Snake Venom on the Blood. With an Appendix* (Melbourne: Stillwell and Co., 1894).

Halford, George B., *On the Injection of Ammonia Into the Circulation* (Melbourne: Stillwell and Knight, 1869).

Hamlin, Christopher, *Cholera: The Biography* (Oxford: Oxford University Press, 2009).

Handley, James, *Mechanical Essays On the Animal Oeconomy* (London: A. Bettesworth and C. Rivington, 1721).

Hansford-Miller, Frank, *Aboriginal and English Medicine in Swan River Colony in 1829* (Willetton: Abcado Publishers, 1990).

Haraway, Donna, *The Companion Species Manifesto: Dogs, People, and Significant Otherness* (Chicago: Prickly Paradigm, 2003).

Hardy, Susan, 'Ferments, zymes and the west wind: adapting disease theories and therapies in New South Wales, 1860–1880', in Harold Attwood and Geoffrey Kenny (eds), *Reflections on Medical History and Health in Australia: Third National Conference on Medical History and Health in Australia 1986* (Melbourne: Medical History Unit, University of Melbourne, 1987), pp. 43–60.

Harré, Rom, *Pavlov's Dog and Schrödinger's Cat: Scenes from the Living Laboratory* (Oxford: Oxford University Press, 2009).

Harris, Henry, *The Birth of the Cell* (New Haven: Yale University Press, 2000).

Hatley, James, 'The uncanny goodness of being edible to bears', in Bruce V. Foltz and Robert Frodeman (eds), *Rethinking Nature: Essays in Environmental Philosophy* (Bloomington: Indiana University Press, 2004), pp. 13–31.

Hatley, James, 'Where the beaver gnaw: predatory space in the urban landscape', in Gary Backhaus and John Murungi (eds), *Transformations of Urban and Suburban Landscapes: Perspectives from Philosophy, Geography, and Architecture* (Lanham: Lexington Books, 2002), pp. 35–53.

Hawgood, Barbara J., 'Doctor Albert Calmette 1863–1933: founder of antivenomous serotherapy and of antituberculous BCG vaccination', *Toxicon*, 37:9 (1999), 1241–58.

Hawgood, Barbara J., 'Pioneers of anti-venomous serotherapy: Dr Vital Brazil (1865–1950)', *Toxicon*, 30:5–6 (1992), 573–9.

Hawgood, Barbara J., 'Sir Charles James Martin MB FRS: Australian serpents and Indian plague, one-hundred years ago', *Toxicon*, 35 (1997), 999–1010.

Hawgood, Barbara J., 'Sir Joseph Fayrer MD FRS (1824–1907) Indian Medical Service: snakebite and mortality in British India', *Toxicon*, 34:2 (1996), 171–82.

Hawgood, Barbara J., 'The life and viper of Dr Patrick Russell MD FRS (1727–1805): physician and naturalist', *Toxicon*, 32:11 (1994), 1295–304.

Heering, Peter, 'An experimenter's gotta do what an experimenter's gotta do – but how?', *Isis*, 101:4 (2010), 794–805.

Higgins, S.B., *Ophidians, Zoological Arrangement of the Different Genera, Including Varieties Known in North and South America, the East Indies, South Africa and Australia* (New York: Boericke & Tafel, 1873).

Hoare, M.E., 'Doctor John Henderson and the Van Diemen's Land Scientific Society', *Records of the Australian Academy of Science*, 1:3 (1966), 7–24.

Hobbins, Peter, 'A spur to atavism: placing platypus poison', *Journal of the History of Biology*, 48:4 (2015), 499–537.

Hobbins, Peter, 'Invasion ontologies: venom, visibility and the imagined histories of arthropods', in Jodi Frawley and Iain McCalman (eds), *Rethinking Invasion Ecologies from the Environmental Humanities* (Oxford: Routledge, 2014), pp. 181–95.

Hobbins, Peter, 'Spectacular serpents: snakebite in colonial Australia', in Jacqueline Healy and Kenneth D. Winkel (eds), *Venom: Fear, Fascination and Discovery* (Melbourne: Medical History Museum, University of Melbourne, 2013), pp. 37–46.

Hobbins, Peter G., 'Serpentine science: Charles Kellaway and the fluctuating fortunes of venom research in interwar Australia', *Historical Records of Australian Science*, 21:1 (2010), 1–34.

Hodgkinson, Clement, *Australia, from Port Macquarie to Moreton Bay; with Descriptions of the Natives, Their Manners and Customs; the Geology, Natural Productions, Fertility, and Resources of That Region* (London: T. and W. Boone, 1845).

Hoffenberg, Peter H., '"A science of our own": nineteenth century exhibitions, Australians and the history of science', in Brett M. Bennett and Joseph M. Hodge (eds), *Science and Empire: Knowledge and Networks of Science across the British Empire, 1800–1970* (Basingstoke: Palgrave Macmillan, 2011), pp. 110–39.

Hogg, G. Heuze, 'On the medicine of the Tasmanian aboriginals', in Gregory Sprott (ed.), *Intercolonial Medical Congress of Australasia. Transactions of the Sixth Session, Held in Hobart, Tasmania, February, 1902* (Hobart: John Vail, 1903), pp. 176–7.

Hooker, Claire, 'Sanitary failure and risk: Pasteurisation, immunisation and the logics of prevention', in Alison Bashford and Claire Hooker (eds), *Contagion: Epidemics, History and Culture from Smallpox to Anthrax* (Annandale: Pluto Press, 2002), pp. 129–49.

Hooker, Claire, and Alison Bashford, 'Diphtheria and Australian public health: bacteriology and its complex applications, c. 1890–1930', *Medical History*, 46:1 (2002), 41–64.

Hüntelmann, Axel C., 'Evaluation as a practical technique of administration: the regulation and standardization of diphtheria serum', in Christoph Gradmann and Jonathan Simon (eds), *Evaluating and Standardizing*

Therapeutic Agents, 1890–1950 (Basingstoke: Palgrave Macmillan, 2010), pp. 31–51.

Hursthouse, Charles, *New Zealand, or Zealandia, the Britain of the South*, vol. I (London: Edward Stanford, 1857).

Huxtable, L. Ralston, 'Snake-bite in Australia – recent statistics and a review of recent observations', in L. Ralston Huxtable (ed.), *Intercolonial Medical Congress of Australasia. Transactions of the Third Session, Held in Sydney, New South Wales, September, 1892* (Sydney: Charles Potter, 1893), pp. 138–54.

Ingold, Tim, 'From trust to domination: an alternative history of human–animal relations', in Aubrey Manning and James Serpell (eds), *Animals and Human Society: Changing Perspectives* (London: Routledge, 1994), pp. 1–22.

Ingold, Tim, 'When ANT meets SPIDER: social theory for arthropods', in Carl Knappett and Lambros Malafouris (eds), *Material Agency: Towards a Non-Anthropocentric Approach* (New York: Springer, 2008), pp. 209–15.

Jamieson, Philip, 'Animal welfare: a movement in transition', in Suzanne Corcoran (ed.), *Law and History in Australia: A Collection of Papers Presented at the 1989 Law and History Conference* (Adelaide: Adelaide Law Review Association, 1991), pp. 21–34.

Jamieson, Philip, 'Duty and the beast: the movement in reform of animal welfare law', *University of Queensland Law Journal*, 16:2 (1991), 238–55.

Jenkins, C.F.H., *The Noah's Ark Syndrome: One Hundred Years of Acclimatisation and Zoo Development in Australia* (Perth: Zoological Gardens Board of Western Australia, 1977).

Johnson, Murray, 'Fangs and faith: the search for an effective antidote against snake envenomation in Australia', *Journal of the Royal Australian Historical Society*, 95:2 (2009), 125–44.

Jonasson, Hermann, *Valedictory Address: The President of the Medical Society of Victoria for the Year 1870* (Melbourne: Stillwell and Knight, 1871).

Jones, Ross L., *Humanity's Mirror: 150 Years of Anatomy in Melbourne* (South Yarra: Haddington Press, 2007).

Keating, Peter, Alberto Cambrosio and Michael Mackenzie, 'The tools of the discipline: standards, models, and measures in the affinity/avidity controversy in immunology', in Adele E. Clarke and Joan H. Fujimura (eds), *The Right Tools for the Job: At Work in Twentieth-Century Life Sciences* (Princeton: Princeton University Press, 1992), pp. 312–54.

Kenny, Robert, *The Lamb Enters the Dreaming: Nathanael Pepper & the Ruptured World* (Melbourne: Scribe, 2007).

Keogh, Luke, '*Duboisia pituri*: a natural history', *Historical Records of Australian Science*, 22:2 (2011), 199–214.

King, William, *An Essay On the Origin of Evil*, 2nd edn, vol. 1 (London: W. Thurlbourn, 1732).

Kippen, Rebecca, 'Rabies in Tasmania', *Chainletter*, 3 (December 2009), 4–5.

Kociumbas, Jan, 'Science as cultural ideology: museums and mechanics' institutes in early New South Wales and Van Diemen's Land', *Labour History*, 64 (1993), 17–33.

Krefft, Gerard, *The Snakes of Australia; An Illustrated and Descriptive Catalogue of All the Known Species* (Sydney: Thomas Richards, 1869).

Kuhn, Thomas S., *The Structure of Scientific Revolutions*, 2nd edn (Chicago: University of Chicago Press, 1970).

Lamb, G., *Specificity of Antivenomous Sera* (Calcutta: Office of the Superintendent of Government Printing, India, 1903).

Lamb, G., and Wm. Hanna, *Standardisation of Calmette's Anti-Venomous Serum with Pure Cobra Venom: The Deterioration of This Serum through Keeping in India* (Calcutta: Office of the Superintendent of Government Printing, India, 1902).

Lamb, George, *Snake-venoms in Relation to Haemolysis* (Calcutta: Office of the Superintendent of Government Printing, India, 1905).

Lansbury, Coral, *The Old Brown Dog: Women, Workers, and Vivisection in Edwardian England* (Madison: University of Wisconsin Press, 1985).

Lassak, E.V., and T. McCarthy, *Australian Medicinal Plants* (North Ryde: Methuen, 1983).

Latour, Bruno, *On the Modern Cult of the Factish Gods*, trans. Catherine Porter and Heather MacLean (Durham: Duke University Press, 2010).

Latour, Bruno, 'On the partial existence of existing and nonexisting objects', in Lorraine Daston (ed.), *Biographies of Scientific Objects* (Chicago: University of Chicago Press, 2000), pp. 247–69.

Latour, Bruno, *The Pasteurization of France*, trans. Alan Sheridan and John Law (Cambridge, Mass.: Harvard University Press, 1988).

Lawrence, Christopher, *Medicine in the Making of Modern Britain, 1700–1920* (London: Routledge, 1994).

Lehane, Robert, *Duelling Surgeon, Colonial Patriot: The Remarkable Life of William Bland* (North Melbourne: Australian Scholarly Publishing, 2011).

Leichhardt, Ludwig, *Journal of an Overland Expedition in Australia, from Moreton Bay to Port Essington, a Distance of Upwards of 3000 Miles, During the Years 1844–1845* (North Adelaide: Corkwood Press, 2000), p. 191.

Leigh, W.H., *Reconnoitering Voyages and Travels, with Adventures in the New Colonies of South Australia* (Milson's Point: Currawong Press, 1982).

Leighton, Mary Elizabeth, and Lisa Surridge, 'The empire bites back: the racialised crocodile of the nineteenth century', in Deborah Denenholz Morse and Martin A. Danahay (eds), *Victorian Animal Dreams: Representations of Animals in Victorian Literature and Culture* (Aldershot: Ashgate, 2007), pp. 249–70.

Lesson, R.-P., *Voyage Autour du Monde Exécuté par Ordre du Roi, sur la Corvette de sa Majesté, La Coquille* (Paris: Arthus Bertrand, 1832).

Liew, Khiun, 'Making health public: English language newspapers and the medical sciences in colonial Malaya (1840s–1941)', *East Asian Science, Technology and Society*, 3:2–3 (2009), 209–29.

Lipitt, Akira Mizuta, *Electric Animal: Toward a Rhetoric of Wildlife* (Minneapolis: University of Minnesota Press, 2008).

Livingstone, David N., *Putting Science in its Place: Geographies of Scientific Knowledge* (Chicago: University of Chicago Press, 2003).

Logan, Cheryl A., 'Before there were standards: the role of test animals in the production of empirical generality in physiology', *Journal of the History of Biology*, 35:2 (2002), 329–63.

Löwy, Ilana, 'On guinea pigs, dogs and men: anaphylaxis and the study of biological individuality, 1902–1939', *Studies in History and Philosophy of Biological and Biomedical Sciences*, 34:3 (2003), 399–423.

Lynch, Michael E., 'Sacrifice and the transformation of the animal body into a scientific object: laboratory culture and ritual practice in the neurosciences', *Social Studies of Science*, 18:2 (1988), 265–89.

Lynn, William S., 'Animals, ethics, and geography', in Jennifer Wolch and Jody Emel (eds), *Animal Geographies: Place, Politics, and Identity in the Nature–Culture Borderlands* (London: Verso, 1998), pp. 280–97.

MacDonald, Donald, *The Bush Boy's Book*, 2nd edn (Sydney: Cornstalk Publishing, 1927).

MacDonald, Helen, 'A scandalous act: regulating anatomy in a British settler colony, Tasmania 1869', *Social History of Medicine*, 20:1 (2007), 39–56.

MacDonald, Helen, *Possessing the Dead: The Artful Science of Anatomy* (Melbourne: Melbourne University Press, 2010).

MacGregor, Arthur, *Animal Encounters: Human and Animal Interaction in Britain from the Norman Conquest to World War One* (London: Reaktion Books, 2012).

Macintyre, Iain, 'George (1830–72) and his son James Hogarth (1863–1941) Pringle: unsung surgical pioneers', *Journal of Medical Biography*, 16:3 (2008), 155–61.

Mackerras, I.M., and Elizabeth N. Marks, 'The Bancrofts: a century of scientific endeavour', *Proceedings of the Royal Society of Queensland*, 84:1 (1973), 1–34.

MacLeod, Roy, 'On visiting the "moving metropolis": reflections on the architecture of imperial science', *Historical Records of Australian Science*, 5:3 (1980), 1–16.

MacLeod, Roy, 'Organizing science under the Southern Cross', in Roy MacLeod (ed.), *The Commonwealth of Science: ANZAAS and the Scientific Enterprise in Australasia, 1888–1988* (Melbourne: Oxford University Press, 1988), pp. 19–39.

Macwhirter, P.J., 'Shifting paradigms: the hard road to acceptance of the contagion principle in Australia', *Australian Veterinary Journal*, 75:7 (1997), 515–19.

Maehle, Andreas-Holger, and Ulrich Tröhler, 'Animal experimentation from antiquity to the end of the eighteenth century: attitudes and arguments', in Nicolaas Rupke (ed.), *Vivisection in Historical Perspective* (London: Croom Helm, 1987), pp. 14–47.

Magendie, François, *Formulary for the Preparation and Employment of Several New Remedies*, 6th edn, trans. Joseph Houlton (London: T. and G. Underwood, 1829).

Malcolmson, Robert, and Stephanos Mastoris, *The English Pig: A History* (London: Hambledon and London, 1998).

Manuel, Diana, 'Marshall Hall (1790–1857): vivisection and the development of experimental physiology', in Nicolaas Rupke (ed.), *Vivisection in Historical Perspective* (London: Croom Helm, 1987), pp. 78–104.

Markwell, Kevin, and Nancy Cushing, 'The "killer of the cane fields": the social construction of the Australian coastal taipan', *Journal of Australian Studies*, 40:1 (2016), 74–91.

Martin, C.J., and A. Calmette, 'Snake-poison and snake-bite', in Thomas Clifford Allbutt (ed.), *A System of Medicine*, vol. 2 (London: MacMillan, 1897), pp. 809–35.

Martin, Jennifer Adams, 'When sharks (don't) attack: wild animal agency in historical narratives', *Environmental History*, 16:3 (2011), 451–5.

Martindale, W. Harrison, and W. Wynn Westcott, *The Extra Pharmacopœia of Martindale and Westcott*, 14th edn (London: H.K. Lewis, 1910).

Mayer, Jed, 'The nature of the experimental animal: evolution, vivisection, and the Victorian environment', in Carol Freeman, Elizabeth Leane and Yvette Watt (eds), *Considering Animals: Contemporary Studies in Human–Animal Relations* (Farnham: Ashgate, 2011), pp. 93–104.

Mazumdar, Pauline M.H., *Species and Specificity: An Interpretation of the History of Immunology* (Cambridge: Cambridge University Press, 1995).

Mazumdar, Pauline M.H., 'The state, the serum institutes and the League of Nations', in Christoph Gradmann and Jonathan Simon (eds), *Evaluating and Standardizing Therapeutic Agents, 1890–1950* (Basingstoke: Palgrave Macmillan, 2010), pp. 118–38.

Mead, Richard, *A Mechanical Account of Poisons, in Several Essays*, 5th (corrected) edn (London: J. Brindley, 1756).

Metcalfe, G., *Australian Zoology* (Sydney: E.W. Cole, 1895).

Miletski, Hani, 'A history of bestiality', in Andrea M. Beetz and Anthony L. Podberscek (eds), *Bestiality and Zoophilia: Sexual Relations with Animals* (Lafayette: Purdue University Press, 2005), pp. 1–22.

Mirtschin, Peter, 'The pioneers of venom production for Australian antivenoms', *Toxicon*, 48:7 (2006), 899–918.

Mitchell, S. Weir, *Researches Upon the Venom of the Rattlesnake: With an Investigation of the Anatomy and Physiology of the Organs Concerned* (Philadelphia: Collins, 1860).

Morison, Patricia, *JT Wilson and the Fraternity of Duckmaloi* (Amsterdam: Editions Rodopi, 1997).

Morus, Iwan Rhys, 'Worlds of wonder: sensation and the Victorian scientific performance', *Isis*, 101:4 (2010), 806–16.

Mueller, A., *On Snake-Poison. Its Action and Its Antidote* (Sydney: L. Bruck, 1893).

Mueller, A., 'Snake-poison; its physical and chemical qualities and physiological action', in L. Ralston Huxtable (ed.), *Intercolonial Medical Congress of Australasia. Transactions of the Third Session, Held in Sydney, New South Wales, September, 1892* (Sydney: Charles Potter, 1893), pp. 155–64.

Mukharji, Projit Bihari, 'Pharmacology, "indigenous knowledge", nationalism: a few words from the epitaph of subaltern science', in Mark Harrison and

Biswamoy Pati (eds), *The Social History of Health and Medicine in Colonial India* (London: Routledge, 2009), pp. 195–212.

Mukharji, Projit Bihari, 'The "cholera cloud" in the nineteenth-century "British world": history of an object-without-an-essence', *Bulletin of the History of Medicine*, 86:3 (2012), 303–32.

Murray, Lisa, 'Old Sydney Burial Ground', *Phanfare: Newsletter of the Professional Historians' Association* (NSW), 228 (January–February 2008), 6–7.

Murrell, William, *What To Do in Cases of Poisoning* (London: HK Lewis & Co., 1921).

Nicholson, Edward, *Indian Snakes. An Elementary Treatise on Ophiology with a Descriptive Catalogue of the Snakes Found in India and the Adjoining Countries* (Madras: Higginbotham & Co., 1870).

Nicholson, Edward, *Indian Snakes. An Elementary Treatise on Ophiology with a Descriptive Catalogue of the Snakes Found in India and the Adjoining Countries*, 2nd edn (Madras: Higginbotham and Co., 1874).

O'Connor, Erin, *Raw Material: Producing Pathology in Victorian Culture* (Durham: Duke University Press, 2000).

Olsen, Penny, *Upside Down World: Early European Impressions of Australia's Curious Animals* (Canberra: National Library of Australia, 2010).

Osborne, W.A., 'George Britton Halford: his life and work', *Medical Journal of Australia*, 1 (1929), 64–71.

O'Sullivan, Siobhan, *Animals, Equality and Democracy* (Basingstoke: Palgrave Macmillan, 2012).

Owen, Charles, *An Essay Towards a Natural History of Serpents* (London: Charles Owen, 1742).

Parker, T. Jeffery, and William A. Haswell, *A Text-book of Zoology*, vol. 2 (London: Macmillan and Co., 1897).

Parnes, Ohad, 'From agents to cells: Theodor Schwann's research notes of the years 1835–1838', in Frederic L. Holmes, Jürgen Renn and Hans-Jörg Rheinberger (eds), *Reworking the Bench: Research Notebooks in the History of Science* (Dordrecht: Kluwer Academic, 2003), pp. 119–39.

Parsonson, Ian, *The Australian Ark: A History of Domesticated Animals in Australia* (Collingwood: CSIRO Publishing, 2000).

Paterson, A.B., 'Johnson's Antidote', in *The Man from Snowy River and Other Verses*, 4th edn (London: Macmillan and Co., 1896), pp. 142–8.

Pearn, John, '"Where there is no doctor": self-help and pre-hospital care in colonial Australia', *Health and History*, 14:2 (2012), 162–80.

Pelling, Margaret, *Cholera, Fever and English Medicine* (Oxford: Oxford University Press, 1978).

Pelling, Margaret, 'The meaning of contagion: reproduction, medicine and metaphor', in Alison Bashford and Claire Hooker (eds), *Contagion: Epidemics, History and Culture from Smallpox to Anthrax* (Annandale: Pluto Press, 2002), pp. 15–38.

Pemberton, Neil, and Michael Worboys, *Mad Dogs and Englishmen: Rabies in Britain, 1830–2000* (Houndmills: Palgrave Macmillan, 2007).

Pemberton, Stephen, 'Canine technologies, model patients: the historical production of hemophiliac dogs in American biomedicine', in Susan Schrepfer and Philip Scranton (eds), *Industrializing Organisms: Introducing Evolutionary History* (New York: Routledge, 2004), pp. 191–213.

Pensabene, T.S., *The Rise of the Medical Practitioner in Victoria* (Canberra: Australian National University, 1980).

Pertzel, Barbara, *For All Creatures: A History of RSPCA Victoria* (Burwood East: RSPCA Victoria, 2006).

Petrow, Stefan, 'Civilizing mission: animal protection in Hobart 1878–1914', *Britain and the World*, 5:1 (2012), 69–95.

Petrow, Stefan, '"Developing the highest moral instincts": protecting animals in Launceston 1879–1906', *History Australia*, 15:3 (2015), 160–82.

Pharmacopœia and Reference Handbook of the Royal Alexandria Hospital for Children, Sydney, 8th edn (Sydney: Australasian Medical Publishing Company, 1951).

Phillips, Gael, 'Snakebite remedies: an historical review of snake bite management in the Australian outback', in John Pearn (ed.), *Outback Medicine: Some Vignettes of Pioneering Medicine* (Brisbane: Amphion Press, 1994), pp. 65–81.

Phillips, Gael, and John Pearn, 'Relict ancient medical practice in Australia', in John Pearn (ed.), *Health, History and Horizons* (Brisbane: Amphion Press, 1992), pp. 347–67.

Pickstone, John V., 'Museological science? The place of the analytical/comparative in nineteenth-century science, technology and medicine', *History of Science*, 32:2 (1994), 112–38.

Pickstone, John V., and Michael Worboys, 'Introduction', *Isis*, 102:1 (2011), 97–101.

Plumwood, Val, 'Human vulnerability and the experience of being prey', *Quadrant*, 39:3 (1995), 29–34.

Proust, A.J., 'Medical care in the colony', in A.J. Proust (ed.), *A Social and Cultural History of Medicine in New South Wales in the 19th Century: Southern Tablelands and Monaro* (Forrest: A.J. Proust, 1999), pp. 39–60.

Prüll, Cay-Rüdiger, 'Paul Ehrlich's standardization of serum: Wertbestimmung and its meaning for twentieth-century biomedicine', in Christoph Gradmann and Jonathan Simon (eds), *Evaluating and Standardizing Therapeutic Agents, 1890–1950* (Basingstoke: Palgrave Macmillan, 2010), pp. 13–30.

Raman, Ramya, Anantanarayanan Raman and P. Ram Manohar, 'The arsenic and mercury-containing Tanjore pills used in treating snake bites in the 18th century Madras presidency', *Current Science*, 106:12 (2014), pp. 1759–63.

Redi, Francesco, *A Letter of Francesco Redi Concerning Some Objections Made Upon His Observations About Vipers Written to Monsieur Bourdelot, Abbott, and Lord of Conde and St. Leger and Monsieur Alexander Morus* (London: John Martyn, 1673).

Reiser, Stanley Joel, *Medicine and the Reign of Technology* (Cambridge: Cambridge University Press, 1978).

Rendle, Richard, *Notes on Snake Bite. Full Directions, What to Do, What to Avoid, and How to Use the Strychnia Antidote, Together With a Description of Queensland Venomous Snakes and How to Distinguish the Venomous from the Harmless*, 2nd edn (Brisbane: Pole, Outridge and Co., 1892).

Rentetzi, Maria, *Trafficking Materials and Gendered Experimental Practices: Radium Research in Early 20th Century Vienna* (New York: Columbia University Press, 2007).

Richards, Stewart, 'Vicarious suffering, necessary pain: physiological method in late nineteenth-century Britain', in Nicolaas Rupke (ed.), *Vivisection in Historical Perspective* (London: Croom Helm, 1987), pp. 125–48.

Richards, Vincent, *The Land-Marks of Snake-Poison Literature, Being a Review of the More Important Researches Into the Nature of Snake-Poisons*, 2nd edn (Calcutta: D.M. Traill, 1885).

Ring, Maree, 'Charles Underwood and his snake bite antidote', *Tasmanian Historical Research Association Papers and Proceedings*, 43:3 (1996), 129–49.

Ritvo, Harriet, 'Animal consciousness: some historical perspective', *American Zoologist*, 40:6 (2000), 847–52.

Ritvo, Harriet, 'Animals in nineteenth-century Britain: complicated attitudes and competing categories', in Aubrey Manning and James Serpell (eds), *Animals and Human Society: Changing Perspectives* (London: Routledge, 1994), pp. 106–26.

Ritvo, Harriet, 'Beasts in the jungle (or wherever)', *Daedalus*, 137:2 (2008), 22–30.

Ritvo, Harriet, 'Border trouble: shifting the line between people and other animals', *Social Research*, 62:3 (1995), 481–500.

Ritvo, Harriet, 'Ordering creation, or maybe not', in Helen Small and Trudi Tate (eds), *Literature, Science, Psychoanalysis, 1830–1970: Essays in Honour of Gillian Beer* (Oxford: Oxford University Press, 2003), pp. 52–63.

Ritvo, Harriet, 'Our animal cousins', *differences: A Journal of Feminist Cultural Studies*, 15:1 (2004), 48–68.

Ritvo, Harriet, *The Animal Estate: The English and Other Creatures in the Victorian Age* (Cambridge, Mass.: Harvard University Press, 1987).

Ritvo, Harriet, *The Platypus and the Mermaid and Other Figments of the Classifying Imagination* (Cambridge, Mass.: Harvard University Press, 1998).

Ritvo, Harriet, 'Zoological nomenclature and the empire of Victorian science', in Bernard Lightman (ed.), *Victorian Science in Context* (Chicago: University of Chicago Press, 1997), pp. 334–53.

Robertson, Muriel, and Keith Inglis, 'Charles James Martin. 9th January 1866–15th February 1955', *Journal of Pathology and Bacteriology*, 71:2 (1956), 519–34.

Rogers, Leonard, *Happy Toil: Fifty-five Years of Tropical Medicine* (London: Frederick Muller, 1950).

Rolls, Eric, *A Million Wild Acres: 200 Years of Man and an Australian Forest* (Melbourne: Thomas Nelson Australia, 1981).

Ross, Karen D., 'Recruiting "friends of medical progress": evolving tactics in the defense of animal experimentation, 1910s and 1920s', *Journal of the History of Medicine and Allied Sciences*, 70:3 (2015), 365–93.

Rountree, Phyllis M., 'The Pasteur Institute and Australia', in Jean Chaussivert and Maurice Blackman (eds), *Louis Pasteur and the Pasteur Institute in Australia* (Kensington: University of New South Wales, 1988), pp. 9–16.

Royal Society for the Prevention of Cruelty to Animals, *Vivisection. Royal Society For the Prevention of Cruelty to Animals and the Royal Commission*, 2nd edn (London: Smith, Elder, & Co., 1876).

Rupke, Nicolaas, 'Introduction', in Nicolaas Rupke (ed.), *Vivisection in Historical Perspective* (London: Croom Helm, 1987), pp. 1–13.

Ryder, Richard D., *Animal Revolution: Changing Attitudes towards Speciesism*, revised edn (Oxford: Berg, 2000).

Schell, Heather, 'Tiger tales', in Deborah Denenholz Morse and Martin A. Danahay (eds), *Victorian Animal Dreams: Representations of Animals in Victorian Literature and Culture* (Aldershot: Ashgate, 2007), pp. 230–48.

Schickore, Jutta, 'Scientists' methods accounts: S. Weir Mitchell's research on the venom of poisonous snakes', in Seymour Mauskopf and Tad Schmaltz (eds), *Integrating History and Philosophy of Science: Problems and Prospects* (Dordrecht: Springer, 2011), pp. 141–61.

Schickore, Jutta, 'Trying again and again: multiple repetitions in early modern reports of experiments on snake bites', *Early Science and Medicine*, 15:6 (2010), 567–617.

Schlegel, H., *Essay on the Physiognomy of Serpents*, trans. Thos. Stewart Traill (Edinburgh: Stewart and Co., 1843).

Selleck, R.J.W., *The Shop: The University of Melbourne 1850–1939* (Carlton: Melbourne University Press, 2003).

Sennert, Daniel, Nicholas Culpeper and Abdiah Cole, *The Sixth Book of Practical Physick of Occult or Hidden Diseases* (London: Peter Cole, 1662).

Shapin, Steven, and Simon Schaffer, *Leviathan and the Air Pump: Hobbes, Boyle, and the Experimental Life* (Princeton: Princeton University Press, 2011).

Shaw, George, *General Zoology; Or Systematic Natural History*, vol. 2, part II (London: G. Kearsley, 1802).

Shaw, George and E.R. Nodder, *Naturalist's Miscellany*, vol. 13 (London: Nodder & Co., 1802).

Shaw, Peter, *A New Practice of Physic*, 7th (corrected) edn, vol. 1 (London: T. and T. Longman, 1753).

Silverstein, Arthur M., *A History of Immunology* (San Diego: Academic Press, 1989).

Simon, Jonathan, 'Monitoring the stable at the Pasteur Institute', *Science in Context*, 21:2 (2008), 181–200.

Simons, John, *The Tiger That Swallowed the Boy: Exotic Animals in Victorian England* (Oxfordshire: Libri Publishing, 2012).

Singh, Dhrub Kumar, '"Clouds of cholera" and clouds around cholera, 1817–70', in Deepak Kumar (ed.), *Disease and Medicine in India: A Historical Overview* (Aligarh: Indian History Congress, 2001), pp. 144–65.

Skabelund, *Aaron Herald, Empire of Dogs: Canines, Japan, and the Making of the Modern World* (Ithaca: Cornell University Press, 2011).

Sneader, Walter, *Drug Discovery: A History* (Chichester: John Wiley & Sons, 2005).

Springthorpe, John William, *Therapeutics, Dietetics and Hygiene: An Australian Text-book* (Melbourne: James Little, 1914).

Sprod, Dan (ed.), *Van Diemen's Land Revealed: Flinders and Bass and Their Circumnavigation of the Island in the Colonial Sloop Norfolk 1798–1799* (Hobart: Blubber Head Press, 2009).

Stanley, Henry M., *How I Found Livingstone: Travels, Adventures and Discoveries in Central Africa: Including an Account of Four Months' Residence with Dr. Livingstone* (London: Samson Low, Marston, Low, and Searle, 1872).

Stark, James F., 'Anthrax and Australia in a global context: the international exchange of theories and practices with Britain and France, c.1850–1920', *Health and History*, 14:2 (2012), 1–25.

Starr, Douglas, *Blood: An Epic History of Medicine and Commerce* (London: Warner Books, 1999).

Stejneger, Leonhard, *The Poisonous Snakes of North America* (Washington: Government Printing Office, 1895).

Stern, Alexandra Minna, 'Yellow fever crusade: US colonialism, tropical medicine, and the international politics of mosquito control, 1900–1920', in Alison Bashford (ed.), *Medicine at the Border: Disease, Globalization and Security, 1850 to the Present* (Houndmills: Palgrave Macmillan, 2006), pp. 41–59.

Stubbe, Henry, *An Epistolary Discourse Concerning Phlebotomy in Opposition to G. Thomson Pseudo-Chymist, a Pretended Disciple of the Lord Verulam* (London, 1671).

Sturm, Christoph Christian, *Reflections for Every Day in the Year, on the Works of God, and of His Providence Throughout All Nature*, 7th edn, vol. 2 (Edinburgh: N.R. Cheyne, 1800).

Swart, Sandra, *Riding High: Horses, Humans and History in South Africa* (Johannesburg: Witwatersrand University Press, 2010).

Tansey, E.M., 'The Wellcome Physiological Research Laboratories 1894–1904: the Home Office, pharmaceutical firms, and animal experiments', *Medical History*, 33:1 (1989), 1–41.

Tauber, Alfred I., and Leon Chernyak, *Metchnikoff and the Origins of Immunology: From Metaphor to Theory* (New York: Oxford University Press, 1991).

Temkin, Owsei, 'The scientific approach to disease: specific entity and individual sickness', in A.C. Crombie (ed.), *Scientific Change: Historical Studies in the Intellectual, Social, and Technical Conditions for Scientific Discovery and Technical Invention, from Antiquity to the Present* (London: Heinemann, 1963), pp. 629–47.

Tench, Watkin, *1788: Comprising a Narrative of the Expedition to Botany Bay and a Complete Account of the Settlement at Port Jackson* (Melbourne: Text Publishing, 1996).

Thompson, C.J.S., *The Mystery and Art of the Apothecary* (London: John Lane The Bodley Head, 1929).

Tidswell, Frank, *Researches on Australian Venoms. Snake-Bite, Snake-Venom and Antivenine. The Poison of the Platypus. The Poison of the Red-Spotted Spider* (Sydney: William Applegate Gullick, 1906).

Todd, Jan, *Colonial Technology: Science and the Transfer of Innovation to Australia* (Cambridge: Cambridge University Press, 2009).

Todd, Jan, 'Science at the periphery: an interpretation of Australian scientific and technological dependency and development prior to 1914', *Annals of Science*, 50:1 (1993), 33–58.

Todd, Jan, 'The Pasteur Institute of Australia – success and failure', in Jean Chaussivert and Maurice Blackman (eds), *Louis Pasteur and the Pasteur Institute in Australia* (Kensington: University of New South Wales, 1988), pp. 25–37.

Topsell, Edward, *The Historie of Serpents* (London: William Jaggard, 1608).

Tribby, Jay, 'Cooking (with) Clio and Cleo: eloquence and experiment in seventeenth-century Florence', *Journal of the History of Ideas*, 52:3 (1991), 417–39.

Turner, Daniel, *De Morbis Cutaneis. A Treatise of Diseases Incident to the Skin*, 5th (corrected) edn (London: R. Wilkin, J. and J. Bonwicke, S. Birt, T. Ward and E. Wicksteed, 1736).

Turner, James, *Reckoning with the Beast: Animals, Pain and Humanity in the Victorian Mind* (Baltimore: Johns Hopkins University Press, 1980).

Tyler, Peter J., 'Our first microbiologist', *Locality* (2001), 10–13.

Victorian Humane Society, *First Annual Report* (Melbourne: Victorian Humane Society, 1875).

Victorian Society for the Prevention of Cruelty to Animals, *Man's Duty To the Lower Animals: Especially Addressed to Victorians* (Melbourne: Mason, Firth & McCutcheon, 1880).

Victorian Society for the Protection of Animals, *A Few Words to Young Australians* (Melbourne: Victorian Society for the Protection of Animals, 1883).

Victorian Society for the Protection of Animals, *Twelfth Annual Report* (Melbourne: Victorian Society for the Protection of Animals, 1883).

Vimieiro Gomes, Ana Carolina, '"Too good to be true": the controversy over the use of permanganate of potash as an antidote to snake poison and the circulation of Brazilian physiology in the nineteenth century', *Bulletin of the History of Medicine*, 86:2 (2012), 152–77.

Waite, Edgar R., *A Popular Account of Australian Snakes With a Complete List of the Species and an Introduction to Their Habits and Organisation* (Sydney: Thomas Shine, 1898).

Walker, R.B., 'Fauna and flora protection in New South Wales, 1866–1948', *Journal of Australian Studies*, 28 (1991), 17–28.

Walker-Meikle, Kathleen, 'Toxicology and treatment: medical authorities and snake-bite in the middle ages', *Korot*, 22 (2013–14), 85–104.

Ward, Samuel, *A Modern System of Natural History*, vol. 11 (London: F. Newbery, 1775–76).

Warner, John Harley, 'The idea of science in English medicine: the "decline of science" and the rhetoric of reform, 1815–45', in Roger French and Andrew

Wear (eds), *British Medicine in an Age of Reform* (London: Routledge, 1991), pp. 136–64.

Webb, Stephen, *Palaeopathology of Aboriginal Australians: Health and Disease Across a Hunter-Gatherer Continent* (Cambridge: Cambridge University Press, 1995).

Weindling, Paul, 'From medical research to clinical practice: serum therapy for diphtheria in the 1890s', in John V. Pickstone (ed.), *Medical Innovations in Historical Perspective* (New York: St Martin's press, 1992), pp. 72–83.

Westrip, Joyce, and Peggy Holroyde, *Colonial Cousins: A Surprising History of Connections Between India and Australia* (Kent Town: Wakefield Press, 2010).

White, John, *Journal of a Voyage To New South Wales With Sixty-Five Plates of Non Descript Animals, Birds, Lizards, Serpents, Curious Cones of Trees and Other Natural Productions* (London: I. Debrett, 1790).

White, Paul S., 'The experimental animal in Victorian Britain', in Lorraine Daston and Gregg Mitman (eds), *Thinking with Animals: New Perspectives on Anthropomorphism* (New York: Columbia University Press, 2005), pp. 59–81.

Wilbert, Chris, 'What is doing the killing? Animal attacks, man-eaters, and shifting boundaries and flows of human–animal relations', in The Animal Studies Group, (eds), *Killing Animals* (Urbana: University of Illinois Press, 2006), pp. 30–49.

Wilkins, John S., *Species: A History of the Idea* (Berkeley: University of California Press, 2009).

Wilkinson, Lise, 'John Hunter and the transmissibility of rabies', *Veterinary History*, 2 (new series 2) (1981–82), 78–84.

Winter, Alison, *Mesmerized: Powers of Mind in Victorian Britain* (Chicago: University of Chicago Press, 1998).

Wittgenstein, Ludwig, *Philosophical Investigations*, 2nd edn, trans. G.E.N. Anscombe (Oxford: Basil Blackwell, 1963).

Wolfe, Cary, 'In the shadow of Wittgenstein's lion: language, ethics, and the question of the animal', in Cary Wolfe (ed.), *Zoontologies: The Question of the Animal* (Minneapolis: University of Minnesota Press, 2003), pp. 1–57.

Wolsterstan, Stanford, *An Enquiry Into the Causes of Diseases in General and the Disturbances of the Humors in Man's Body Wherein the Nature of the Blood, of the Air and of a Pestilential Constitution Are Briefly Considered* (London: Thomas Basset, 1692).

Worboys, M., 'British colonial medicine and tropical imperialism: a comparative perspective', in A.M. Luyendijk-Elshout *et al.* (eds), *Dutch Medicine in the Malay Archipelago, 1816–1942* (Amsterdam: Rodopi, 1989), pp. 153–67.

Worboys, Michael, *Spreading Germs: Disease Theories and Medical Practice in Britain, 1865–1900* (Cambridge: Cambridge University Press, 2000).

Worboys, Michael, 'Vaccine therapy and laboratory medicine in Edwardian Britain', in John V. Pickstone (ed.), *Medical Innovations in Historical Perspective* (New York: St Martin's Press, 1992), pp. 84–103.

Yapp, Brunsdon and Wilma George, 'Other animals', in Wilma George and Brunsdon Yapp (eds), *The Naming of Beasts: Natural History in the Medieval Bestiary* (London: Duckworth, 1991), pp. 190–202.

Zinsser, Hans, *Infection and Resistance: An Exposition of the Biological Phenomena Underlying the Occurrence of Infection and the Recovery of the Animal Body from Infectious Disease* (New York: The Macmillan Company, 1914).

INDEX

Notes: page numbers in italics refer to illustrations; 'n.' after a page reference indicates the number of a note on that page; legislation is listed under the short name of respective Acts.